MYBYBLE

FOR THE EXTENDED LIFESPAN

Carole Lynn Steiner
嘉露蓮

Copyright © 2014 by Carole Lynn Steiner.

Library of Congress Control Number: 2014904202
ISBN: Hardcover   978-1-4931-7457-7
              Softcover   978-1-4931-7458-4
              eBook   978-1-4931-8129-2

All rights reserved. No part of this book may be reproduced or transmitted in any form or by any means, electronic or mechanical, including photocopying, recording, or by any information storage and retrieval system, without permission in writing from the copyright owner.

Any people depicted in stock imagery provided by Thinkstock are models, and such images are being used for illustrative purposes only.
Certain stock imagery © Thinkstock.

This book was printed in the United States of America.

Rev. date: 04/11/2014

To order additional copies of this book, contact:
Xlibris LLC
1-888-795-4274
www.Xlibris.com
Orders@Xlibris.com
540209

TABLE OF CONTENTS

Dedication 9
Disclaimer 11
Information That is Key to Mybyble 11
Learn 13
Tips, Tips, and More Tips! 18
Sex and Coconut Oil or Emu Oil :
    Vaginal Dryness, Penile Lubrication 22
Face and Neck Moisturizers:
    Skin Care (and for Thyroid Gland and Eyebrows), Massage 24
Washing the Face, Removing Makeup 25
Hair Regrowth and Color Restoration 26
Peyronie's Disease (Crooked or Curved Penis) 28
Coconut or Emu Oil For Babies' and Children's Derrières;
    Buttock, Anal, and Rectal Distress 29
Burn Marks, Age Spots 29
Soap 30
Body Movements to Relieve Pain, Ease Tired Feet,
    Fix Hip, Adjust Jaw, Lift Rib Cage, Correct Shoulders
    and Posture, Elongate Spine 31
Elongate the Spine While Sitting 37
Lengthen/Strengthen the Neck 38
Firm the Chin 38
Wrinkles, Expressions: Mirror, Mirror on the Wall 38
Frowning 39
Clench Your Fist to Remember 39
If You are Tall, Don't Shrink 39
Scoliosis: One Shoulder Lower than the Other 40
Food Combining Weight, Gas, Bloating, Digestive Problems 42
Weight Loss, Weight Control, Diet: The Body Needs
    Good Fats, Whole Foods, and Not Fractionated Foods 44
Drink Warm Water 46

Probiotics for Gums and Periodontal Disease:
    'Pulling' for Gum Health 47
Probiotics: Getting Rid of that Paunch and Some Inches 49
Goat's Milk: Cow's Milk is Meant For Baby Cows 50
Hum for Healthy Vocal Cords..51
Flashlight Uses..52
Short-Term Memory Loss...54
Hang Upside Down or, at Least, Partially Inverted: Back Issues,
    Digestion, Circulation, Brain and Eye Nourishment, Skin............54
Back Discomfort 57
Close Your Eyes in Order to Focus:
    Wiggle the Toothbrush, Visualization...58
Distilled Water for Cleaning Spots 59
Distilled Water Information 61
Digestion/Indigestion Nutrition 61
    Hydrochloric Acid, Digestive Enzymes..61
    Digestive Enzymes..62
    Tips for Better Digestion...62
    What Digestive Supplements Do I Take? 64
    How Do I Know If I Have Too Little Stomach Acid? 66
Exercises/Toning: For Which You Do Not Need To Buy Equipment 67
    Back of Arms (Underarm Flab) 67
    Eyes..68
    Neck and Face...69
Funny Bone (Elbow) and Isometrics:
    Nerve Damage, Weak Muscles, Tendons and Ligaments,
    Improved Bustline and Thighs, Used in Scoliosis Treatment........70
Rebounding on Minitrampoline 72
Cross Crawl: Memory, Coordination,
    Brain Function, Mental Agility, Balance 74
    What is Cross Crawl?..75
Walking Backward: Tone the Abdomen 77
    Walking Forward...77
    Stair Climbing...78
Heart Palpitations, Arrhythmias: Cough to Get Your Heart Beating 78
    Restless Leg Syndrome...78
Urine to the Rescue:
    Cuts, Paper Cuts, Insect Bites, Rashes, Hives, Rosacea................83

Deep Breathing:
  Cleanse System, Expel Polluted Air, Tone Cells, Hot Flashes 86
Frozen Bread or Cake 87
Distilled Water 88
Self-Tanning Lotions: Surgical Rubber Gloves to the Rescue 88
Protect Nails and Hands: Packing, Cleaning,
  Chores, Grocery Shopping: Use Surgical (Rubber) Gloves 89
Removing Nail Polish 89
Fur 89
Lipstick on Teeth 90
Collectibles 90
Nail Fungus: Fingers and Toes; Cuticle Infection 90
Protecting Pantyhose 92
Absorbent Cotton 92
How to Brush One's Teeth 93
Toothbrushes, Colds, Bacteria, Viruses 93
Good-Gums for Healthy Brushing of Teeth:
  Use Celtic Sea Salt in Water to Flush the Mouth All Day Long 94
Celtic Sea Salt with Food; Good Salt Critical for Good Health 95
Floss with Floss Sticks 96
Peroxide: Teeth, Gums, Sore Throat, Moles, Fungus 96
Chopsticks? No! Future Sticks! 97
Skin: Moisturize, Freshen 99
Moisturize 99
  Men and Women 99
  Drink 99
  Spray 101
  Cream/Oil 101
  Men 103
Makeup Base 103
Cream Eye Shadow and Cheek Blush (Rouge) 104
Buffing Skin or Face 105
  Towel 106
  Soap 106
Stockings, Pantyhose, Varicose Veins, Spider Veins:
  Support for Impaired Circulation 106
Perfume or Men's Cologne Or Aftershave:
  Use Petroleum Jelly (Vaseline or House Brand) 108
Camouflage Flaws 108

Eyelid Irritation 109
Heat—or Cold—Treatment: Injuries, Muscle Pain, Joint Pain 110
Ear Pressure, Airplanes 110
Eye Makeup 111
Sleep Facts and Sleeping Positions:
    Face Wrinkles, Backache, Circulation, Venous Insufficiency 111
Eye Makeup Brushes 114
Technique for Using Eye Creams/Moisturizing:
    Toning Skin Around the Eyes 114
Bowel, Stool, Elimination, Constipation,
    Babies And Potties, Support for Bladder 115
Saliva, Nail Polish 118
Chipping Nail Polish 119
Saliva and Urine Contain Healing Enzymes:
    Stop A Run in Stockings / Pantyhose with Saliva 119
Hot Flashes 120
    Breathe 120
    Herbs And Legume 120
Fish Oil for Health (And Even Hot Flashes, Inflammation, Stroke
    Prevention) 121
Fish Oil and Vitamin A: Cracks on the Heels—Both on
    the Inner Side of the Heel and on the Outside of the Heel 122
Danger of Low-Fat/No-Fat Diets:
    Strokes, Dandruff, Flaking in Eyebrows, Cracks in Skin 125
Good Fats, Healthy Fats 126
Colds, Coughs, Sore Throats:
    Hair Dryer (Great for During Pregnancy), Supplements 128
Veterinarian Products, Animals 130
Clearing Sinuses: The Ultimate Solution 131
    Breathing Bad Air, Rash on Face or Body,
    Beginning of A Cold 131
How to Gargle (Especially for Sore Throats) 133
Gargles: Sore Throat, Overused Voice 133
Honey and Apple Cider Vinegar: Coughs, Colds,
    Bladder Problems, Kidney Problems, Urination Problems 134
Nodules on Vocal Cords: Strained Voice, Overused Voice 136
Teeth, Gums, Dentists 137
Collagen or Juvéderm Injections 137
"Don't Pick!"—And Other Bon Mots From Mom 138

Horseradish: Stomach, Liver, General Health 139
Hangover? A Little Too Much Alcohol?
    Stomach Sick? Poisoning From Food or Other? Overdose? 139
Are Pots and Pans Poisoning You?: Nausea, Chest Pain/
    Constriction, Inexplicable Rash, Eyebrows Curling 140
Dandruff, Dry Hair after Shampoo 142
Chill It! Icing Wine 142
Recorking an Open Bottle of Wine 143
Sleep Problems, Insomnia, Restless Legs 143
Venous Insufficiency, Circulation, Hemorrhoids:
    Tone Inner Thighs and Buttocks (See End of Article) 146
Food Store / Supermarket / Any Store Checkout: Beware Of Germs 151
Tea and Loose Leaf Tea 151
    How to Prepare Tea 152
Washing Fruits and Vegetables:
    Never Antibacterial Soaps or Wipes 154
Pillows and Teddy Bears: Eliminate Dust Mites Using Cold Air 155
Watering Plants, Gardening with Hydrogen Peroxide! 155
Stress 156
Full-Spectrum Lightbulbs—Natural Lighting 157
Proof that Consistent Diet and Supplements Work 158
Cervical Dysplasia: What Started Carole Lynn
    on the Road to Natural Health Care? 159
Investing, Margin 166
The Extended Lifespan, and are you Prepared for it Financially? 168
Investing: How to Interview an Investment Advisor 169
    The Broker 169
    The Portfolio 170
Source List—Assembled by Category and not Alphabetically 171
Index 181
Author's Biography 189

DEDICATION

To my parents, Caroline and Bill, who created me and brought me up with total love and kindness and taught me to be diligent, to laugh, and to reach out. When I started working, they also told me, "Carole, you must stop smiling so much and being so nice to everyone. People mistake niceness for stupidity." A few years later, my Mom apologized (the only time ever) for that and told me that being just who I am makes me special. Then I met my darling Murray, who firmly supported my belief in healthy living while he gradually rewired my brain to function on a whole new level in business and into the thinking body that I am today. I wish you, dear reader, what I wish for myself: That the second half of our lives is the best half!

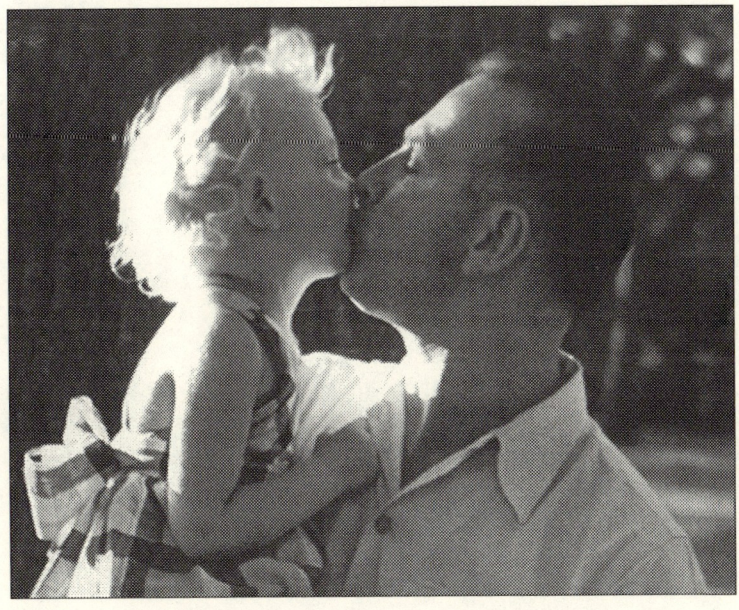

This is my Daddy . . . with his Carole Lynn at age 3!

Disclaimer

Everything about which I write pertains to what *I* do. Any products or methods are what *I* buy or do and what are beneficial for *me*. I am happy to write about my successes with various things and what I have done for others. This is my experience.

For people taking prescription drugs, one must be careful regarding adding supplements while taking those drugs. For example, vitamin K2 would not go well with blood thinners. One should check with one's doctor for contraindications as well as reading online about such issues.

This book is not intended to provide medical advice. Neither the author nor publisher take responsibility for any consequences from any treatment, procedure, exercise, dietary modification, action, or application which results from reading or following the information contained in this book. The publication of this information does not constitute the practice of medicine, and this information does not replace the advice of your physician or other health care provider. The author and publisher disclaim any liability, loss, or risk incurred, directly or indirectly, as a result of the use and application of the contents of this publication. If you are unwilling to be bound by this disclaimer, you should not buy this publication.

Information that Is Key to *Mybyble*

Three decades of continuously and diligently reading medical research, health newsletters, and articles—as well as originally talking with the brilliant Dr. Linus Pauling and his incredible Medical Director, Dr. Ewan Cameron, and being encouraged by them to pursue my interests in natural health care—contribute to this vast and always growing knowledge base. If you ask me why I wrote something, the direct answer is "Because I say so. Because I have read this, learned this, or used this."

I have simplified certain information and provided wording that is understandable to the reader; detailed medical information is not provided. Where a topic piques further interest, there is a wealth of information online.

There is a "Source List" at the end of *Mybyble*. For every article where a product is mentioned, I will provide the name of the company from which I purchase that product and its contact data. **Personally,**

I abhor reading articles where a product is mentioned yet not the name of the manufacturer. I also indicate which sources provide sales and promotions and offer other benefits to customers.

Here and there I repeat a tip or advisement because it is pertinent to not one article but to two. Any mention of *drinking water* means pure water without fluoride or chlorine. In most cities, this indicates bottled water. Be sure to check the provider and know that the water comes from deep wells. You do *not* want bottled municipal water. Read labels!

I have received no compensation from any of the companies mentioned.

In everything I write, I will explain <u>*why*</u> I make a specific comment. It is so very annoying to read or hear "Don't do this" or "Do this" without the specific explanation of <u>WHY</u> and learning what is behind the concept.

"What Started Carole Lynn on the Road to Natural Health Care?" is toward the end of *Mybyble* **in the article "Cervical Dysplasia".**

Dear reader, do not feel overwhelmed with the information in some articles. Reread them. Make notes. Then come back to them in a few days. Rereading is clarifying. **Do not look at this as work but as effort to improve the body as one looks toward** *the extended lifespan* **and the burdens placed upon the individual for coping with issues that rarely existed when the lifespan was much shorter. Everything that one does in order to improve health is not work but necessary <u>effort</u>! It takes effort to stay healthy into one's nineties, and every little improvement contributes to that goal.**

Learn

Many things that occur in and on our bodies are <u>symptoms</u> which can be treated successfully. They are <u>not</u> end results. If you glue a cracked plate, you still have a crack. You must learn to look at what your body tells you and ask why. Drugs most often do **not** treat the underlying condition that **caused** the symptom (for example, palpitations, ministroke, prematurely graying hair, lower back pain) in particular because the diagnosis is incorrect. Too many diagnoses go straight for prescription drugs to stop the symptom rather than finding out **why** the symptom occurred.

Persistent sniffles and clogged sinuses cannot be cured with over-the-counter nose spray. Missing bowel movements—or many of them—cannot be cured with laxatives. Twitches, palpitations, dandruff, brittle/peeling nails, and cracks on heels of the feet are all symptoms.

Take control of your health. It takes considerable effort. You must look things up in alternative (what I call <u>natural</u>) medicine books. *Prescription for Nutritional Healing* by Dr. James F. Balch is a good, all-inclusive reference book. It is a start.

Rodale Press (the group that publishes *Prevention* magazine) used to publish several informative books: *The Complete Book of Vitamins* (1984), *The Complete Book of Minerals for Health* (1972), and *The Right Dose: How to Take Vitamins and Minerals Safely* (1987). They can now be sourced online and wherever old books are carried and are worth having on hand as reference books. They are thick tomes with a wealth of information and can educate the reader. If you purchase them or borrow them from the library, I suggest having a large notepad. You will want to take copious notes.

In my opinion, though, **more important in the long run than the books** (albeit those are excellent in providing the reader with a detailed commentary on supplements/nutrients) **are the following newsletters**, because they arrive daily via e-mail (except for *Health Alert*), are **current** (including news on new products) and **accessible**, and—<u>*read as a group*</u>—offer varied and significant health information. There are several excellent newsletters, which I read, that are **written by doctors who show that there are natural ways to approach and understand health issues. Reading them is an ongoing education for my whole body.**

All—except Dr. West—offer these complimentary daily health e-mails. You should definitely sign up. Additionally, Dr. Mercola offers the most incredible, in-depth daily e-mails on many health topics, including an archive of past articles and news.

When one subscribes to those newsletters that are mailed through the post office and for which there is an annual fee, one also receives a myriad of complimentary brochures which do have value in educating you. Additionally, during the year, some of these newsletters offer special annual subscription pricing. You will be alerted if you are an e-mail subscriber. If you are a **new** subscriber, do not hesitate to ask if there is a special rate at that time.

The newsletters (both through e-mail and the post office) are the following:

>The www.mercola.com newsletter (toll-free US number: 877-985-2695) which is only via e-mail and is complimentary. Sign up online. *Personal Note:* I cannot begin to enumerate the many tips that I receive from reading Mercola.com, especially for one's health and that of the environment (for example, the pesticides and fungicides killing off our bees). I credit Dr. Mercola in articles in *Mybyble*; for example, in the article on hip health and a maneuver that fixed my hip!
>
>**Health Alert** newsletter comes via the post office, is written by Dr. Bruce West, DC, and has NO advertising! If you want to **learn about <u>which</u> supplements to take** for various health problems, **this** is the newsletter for you! Dr. West recommends the **Standard Process products which are whole food-based**! Some are described in *Mybyble*. The *subscription includes, at this time, a written*

consultation with Dr. West after you complete a health profile. If one has any concern regarding **heart disease or cancer**, certainly consult with Dr. West. He has considerable history using whole food-based supplements for various conditions. *Personal Note:* It is Dr. West who has educated me—through *Health Alert*—regarding the importance of treating the **cause** and not the symptom. For example, do not treat the clogged sinus or sniffle (with a nose spray, for example); treat what is *causing* the clog or sniffle. Do not treat the palpitation but find and treat what is causing the heart to flutter (skip beats). See the *Mybyble* article "Heart Palpitations, Arrhythmias". I learned that one cannot cure anything with synthetic products (www.healthalert.com).

Nutrition and Healing from Dr. Jonathan V. Wright. One can sign up online for the complimentary e-mail at www.wrightnewsletter.com/etips/freecopy.html. There is also the subscription newsletter with a 50 percent discount for those at least age 60. Dr. Wright is well known also for establishing his Tahoma Clinic and for being a pioneer in **holistic medicine** and **bio-identical hormone replacement therapy**. *Personal Note:* Aside from regular solid articles, it is excellent to have access to the Tahoma Clinic and to learn about bio-identical hormones.

"Health Sciences Institute": Sign up for the newsletter at www.hsionline.com. The toll-free number is 888-213-0764. This newsletter comes through the mail and has an annual fee. One can also receive HSI's complimentary daily e-mail, HSI e-Alert. Sign up online. HSI informs the reader about new products and indicates where to buy them (usually from the manufacturer) and often with a discount to those who are HSI members. *Personal Note:* I always have read that most toothpastes are useless in contributing to the health of the teeth and are dangerous as well (notice that the labels warn people **not** to swallow[!], and, if a child swallows what covers the toothbrush [especially if it contains fluoride], to "call poison control"). Primarily, this is because most toothpastes have chemical ingredients as well as fluoride (not good—one never wants to swallow toxic substances) and glycerin *(which coats the teeth and prevents them from remineralizing!)*. One day I am reading my "Health Sciences Institute" subscription newsletter (January 2012, vol. 16, no. 7), and there is the article on **"Good-Gums"**. I finally found this **all-natural powder—minus any chemicals—and safe even if some is swallowed**. I was especially impressed because it contains gray sea salt, which, as I know, safely cleans teeth, refreshes breath, and improves gum health. *Please read about Good-Gums in* Mybyble.

The other wonderful product that I learned about here is for **circulation, venous insufficiency, and hemorrhoids**, all of which are related to one's veins. It is DiosVein. *Please read about DiosVein under "Venous Insufficiency, Circulation, Hemorrhoids"* in Mybyble.

Daily Dose with William Campbell Douglass II, MD. One can sign up for the complimentary e-mail at http://www.douglassreport.com/dailydose/freecopy.html. The toll-free number is 888-213-0685. There is also the subscription newsletter with a 50 percent discount for those at least age 60. *Personal Note:* Many years ago I suffered from terrible **pain in my lower back**. Whether getting up from bed in the morning or rising from a seat at the theater, my back was *so* stiff! I consulted with every type of doctor to no avail. One day I was reading the newsletter that Dr. Douglass at that time wrote ("Second Opinion"), and he wrote about lower-back pain, saying that before you go and try all kinds of medical things, you should take **vitamin D3**. He indicated that often lower-back pain can be a ***symptom*** of a **vitamin D deficiency**. Please understand that—at that time—no one was talking or writing about vitamin

D3. He was the first doctor from whom I read any such comments. I immediately purchased these tablets, and, to my amazement, within a few days the stiffness was easing up, and within a few weeks my back was perfect. *Please see the complete article "Back Discomfort" here in* Mybyble.

There is a single-page complimentary health e-mail from Nan Kathryn Fuchs, PhD ("Dr. Nan"). It is "Women's Health Alert". Sign up at www.womenshealthletter.com for the health alert *e-mail* which, I find, presents some very good articles. Note that there is also a subscription newsletter, so select the right item when signing up.

True, all except Dr. West advertise various items in flyers enclosed with the subscription newsletters and mentioned in the complimentary e-mail letters (note: I do *not* purchase any of their vitamins or minerals); however, their articles can be excellent. **Read as a group**, you will learn a great deal and gradually feel confident in taking control of your health, not running to doctors or hospitals for everything, and **you will understand your body**.

I have been learning for thirty years. Nothing debilitating is naturally attributed to aging. **Growing up, we need certain nutrients to grow successfully. Aging, we need particular supplements in order to age gracefully and remain healthy.**

From these newsletters—both subscription and complimentary—**I have been more than repaid (over these many years)** with healthier back, gums, circulation, and total health, a confidence in the knowledge that I gain, and much more. **I believe that you can use *Mybyble* to your benefit in the same way. Any great tip that lasts a lifetime allows the reader to reap a great reward**, and *Mybyble* has many such tips all in one slender digest. It opens paths for you, dear reader.

Tips, Tips, and More Tips!

Clear your palate of spicy or hot seasoning with <u>bread</u>! Water or liquid will not do it. Bread will absorb the offending seasoning, and one can either expectorate (spit it out) or swallow it.

Always keep some soft bread available. If a **bone catches in the throat**, soft bread will capture it and carry it down and out.

Freezing foods? Use plastic bags from the supermarket produce department; double-bag the item; and freeze breads, cakes, leftovers, coffee beans, flaxseeds, almost anything. The <u>double</u>-bag effect really protects the food. Label the bag with a sticky note, or keep an inventory list so you know what you have.

Your facial skin is so delicate. **Use the washcloth** gently. Instead of circular motions forward, go **backward** counterclockwise (which is a milder motion), and use your <u>nondominant</u> hand for a still gentler touch. Never stretch skin by rubbing or scrubbing. Over the years, mistreatment will cause trouble. Damage is cumulative.

Applying makeup: For a light touch, dab on with pinky or ring finger (use the least forceful finger) or middle finger. **Patting on makeup or moisturizer with a nondominant finger** will prevent injuring delicate skin over the long term.

*Keep stockings / **pantyhose in the freezer**.* This can extend the life span (by preventing runs). If you keep a large inventory of hose, just put one of each shade in the freezer.

Packing/unpacking on a trip? Undressing when you get home from work? Undoing your briefcase? Supermarket shopping? **Wear surgeons' rubber gloves** (the thin ones), and **protect your polished nails**! Buy them in Home Depot, Lowe's, or a surgical supply store in quantity. Aside from white and clear, I have even found them in turquoise blue! They make a statement when you are shopping.

Using a **bandage** on sensitive skin? Do you think that it will hurt too much when pulled off at a later time? Remove some of the adhesive by sticking it to a clean sink or tile wall and pulling it off once, twice, or thrice in order to remove some adhesive. Then it will not be so difficult to pull off your tender skin at a later time. Children will giggle or laugh when they see you do this and not worry so much about having that bandage put on.

Put cotton balls in your ears when using a hair dryer. **Protect your hearing!**

If you read the newspapers in a restaurant and also drink tea, note that leftover tea will easily remove **newsprint from your fingers** and <u>not</u> dry out your skin (which the soaps in many restrooms do). Just get a paper towel from the restroom and dab it into the remaining tea (even if it has milk in it). Rub your fingers to remove the newsprint while leaving your skin smooth.

Use a couple of drops of NutriBiotic Grapefruit Seed Extract (from organically grown grapefruit and unfiltered; see "Source List") on **raw oysters or clams**. Allow them to sit for a few minutes in order to **kill bacteria**. There is little taste from the GSE, especially when you use cocktail sauce or horseradish. Also, when you are **drinking water** (anywhere worldwide) and you have concern about its **purity**, place six to fifteen drops (and stir to disperse it) in that table water in order to protect yourself.

If you use **toothpicks**, soak them in 3 percent hydrogen peroxide, allow them to dry, and then have a better implement to clean between teeth and on gums.

The best treatment for **pimples** that I have found is **3 percent hydrogen peroxide**. Use a toothpick (or similar slender implement) or a Q-tip to dot the peroxide onto the blemish. I have found that peroxide stops a pimple 'in its tracks'. If the blemish is slightly open, the liquid may sting a little and even turn the spot white. This lasts briefly. (*Read further in* Mybyble *about other treatments for* **skin rashes** *and pimples, including urine and Retin-A.*)

Keep **silver jewelry** in silver bags (those that you use for silverware). It saves you from having to polish your jewelry due to tarnish.

Keep **earrings** in a pouch that is stitched down the middle. There are two separate interior spaces keeping the earrings from clunking together. If you do not want to take the time to stitch a pouch, simply use two small safety pins down the middle in order to create two compartments.

Filing nails: Some years ago, a manicurist told my mother (who told me): "File your nails **before** removing the polish, because this protects the nails and gives them support from the abrasiveness of the emery board or file."

Posture: Do not slump! Meaning keep your shoulders, back, and chest held up when standing, walking, or sitting. This will tighten the abdomen and stomach which, in turn, will provide support for the back. Good posture will reward you in later years. (*Much more on this in* Mybyble*, including __how__ to have good posture.*)

Perfume or men's cologne: Use a sheer dab of petroleum jelly on wrists and behind the ears. Put your perfume or cologne over it. The **fragrance will last much longer** than when put only on the skin.

Opening an English muffin: Use the tines of a fork. They make a nice, fluffy interior, which toasts so well.

Dry nail polish by holding fingers by vents of an air-conditioner blowing cold. I use sixty-four degrees; the polish is dry within a couple of minutes. Hum while drying the nails. See *Mybyble* article "Hum for Healthy Vocal Cords".

BURNS: *Ice is used for burns.* Keep ice packs (both small and medium sized) in the freezer for those kitchen-burn emergencies. Never put butter or grease on a burn. It is ice that will prevent or ameliorate blisters. Additionally, once the pain from the burn has subsided due to the application of ice packs (or putting ice cubes into a plastic bag or clean cotton towel and placing that on the burn), you can dab on George's Always Active® Aloe Vera (see "Source List"). Aloe is a soothing ingredient for burns. You may need to do this a number of times depending upon the burn.

MYBYBLE

Personal Note: Some years ago, I was at someone's home for a party. The man's mother was in the kitchen frying chicken, and the grease caught on fire. Foolishly, she tried to get the pan to the sink while her son was trying to grab the burning pan. It fell, and the flaming oil went all over his right foot (as he was casually not wearing shoes). The screams brought us all running. As soon as I saw the disaster, I grabbed a clean wastebasket, made the man sit down, put his foot into the basket, and then piled ice cubes from the bar onto his foot. Good thing that this was a party and there were lots of ice cubes. His mother kept yelling to put butter on while I stuck with ice. She finally convinced her son to use butter, and the minute that he did, he was in excruciating pain and went back into the ice. They called their doctor who said: "Get him to the hospital immediately, and I will meet you there. And keep that foot packed in ice!" Later, at the hospital, the doctor told them that my quick action with ice saved this man's foot.

A few years ago, I stupidly heated a cup of water in the microwave in my office in order to make tea. As I removed the cup, the water erupted and spewed scalding liquid over the top of my right hand. I kept that hand in ice for five hours before the pain was gone. I never had a blister. I mention "Burns" elsewhere in *Mybyble*.

TAKING A PILL: When trying to swallow pills, most people tilt the head and neck <u>back</u>. In fact, one should tilt the chin a bit <u>forward</u> which gives a more natural swallowing position. Try it—with one pill in the mouth—and see.

*Life after death? Do NOT save **discontinued items***: Sometime back, they said that some country was pointing missiles toward the United States and that they would probably hit New York or Washington, D.C. What was my first thought? "Carole, you may as well use up all your favorite **DISCONTINUED lipstick colors** that you have been saving and using so sparingly! You cannot take them with you!"

Hydrate the body: <u>**A symptom of the body needing water is when the corners of the mouth seem to sweat.**</u> You actually go to dab at the corners because they seem to be damp; however, nothing is there. It is a symptom of dehydration. So is a **hard stool**.

21

White **spots on fingernails, dandruff,** and **flaking in eyebrows and by eyelashes** can be **symptoms** of zinc—as well as fats—deficiency. See *"Danger of Low-Fat / No-Fat Diet"*.

Remember to LAUGH! A hearty laugh is good for your heart and body. And, as told to me and attributed to Confucius: "People with the greatest capacity for laughter have the greatest intelligence!" (In which case, we laughers must be geniuses.)

SEX and COCONUT OIL or EMU OIL
Vaginal Dryness, Penile Lubrication

Over the years, women—as well as men—have asked me what to use for **vaginal lubrication (or for lubricating the penis** whether with or without a condom). There are two perfect products which are 100 percent natural. They have NO chemicals, and to me, that is the key statement. I do not want to use anything internally (whether vaginally or in my mouth) that has chemicals in it! Which product works best for you depends upon your preferences. These products are natural and nontoxic, and they are the perfect **lubricant when making love.** They have the **added bonus of being edible!**

The two companies and products are the following (*there is more about both products in* Mybyble *article "Face and Neck Moisturizers: Skin Care"*):

> ***Thunder Ridge Emu Oil***: The oil is from the largest nonflying bird. Vast information is available online. The use of emu oil goes back centuries. This deep-penetrating oil has anti-aging, anti-inflammatory, moisturizing, and healing properties.
>
> ***Omega Nutrition's Organic Virgin Coconut Oil:*** There is a wealth of information available online on the benefits of coconut oil. In particular, the fats and proteins it contains moisturize the skin both internally and externally, and three of the fats are antimicrobial.

It is the lauric acid that has the properties of being antibacterial, antiviral, and anti-acne.

Both products have a milky, gel-like consistency. For sexual relations, I prefer emu oil, and those for whom I have recommended either product tend to prefer the emu in this particular category because it has a more gel-like substance whereas the coconut oil changes its consistency according to the weather (going from a firm substance to an oil consistency). Depending upon the outdoor temperature and humidity, coconut oil changes its viscosity. It can be solid (not hard, just a firm gel) or a loose oil. It is always funny to me that even though my home is air-conditioned in summer and heated in winter, it is the prevailing outdoor weather and humidity which affect coconut oil's appearance.

Both products are antimicrobial and thus antibacterial, antifungal, and antiviral, and they are **stable at room temperature**; they can be kept (handy) in the bedroom and can be introduced into the body as a safe ingredient compared to chemical lubricants. There is no danger if either product gets into the mouth.

Emu oil and coconut oil are natural easers for sexual intercourse anytime and certainly at the times of one's life when nature needs a boost. Dabbed around and into the vagina and onto the penis (and also onto condoms; just be sure that the particular condom material does not deteriorate, although this would be unexpected, especially since organic, cold-pressed coconut oil and also emu oil are edible), **they are a natural lubricant.**

I suggest that you try one product for a week and then the other. That is really a pleasurable chore.

Please note that you **never refrigerate** these products. They are kept at room temperature. They do not go rancid. Hence, when used anywhere on the skin, they can work beneficially in order to enhance moisture and skin condition. The fact that a product can remain in perfect condition at room temperature (as does raw honey) tells you that it is pure as well as antimicrobial.

Vaginal maintenance: One can also introduce emu oil or coconut oil into the vagina nightly (just before going to sleep). Be sure to gently push it well in so that it coats all the internal walls. It moisturizes the internal skin and penetrates deeply through layers of skin, and over time, emu oil can reinvigorate vaginal moisture and health.

Other sections of *Mybyble* will describe other benefits of these wondrous nutrient oils which have been used for thousands of years— no chemicals added!

FACE AND NECK MOISTURIZERS
SKIN CARE (and for Thyroid Gland and Eyebrows), MASSAGE

Guess what two products return at the other end of the spectrum? . . . I mean, body. Coconut oil and emu oil. They are the finest natural nutrients for the face, neck, and scalp, and they are **noncomedogenic** (they **do not clog pores**).

They are the most wonderful nighttime products for **really penetrating and producing results**. And it would be **hard to beat the price**. There are some very significant skin products that have used small amounts of these oils in their costly ones. Now you can acquire these products as 100 percent pure and **not** diluted with chemicals or other ingredients.

I believe in alternating their use. Sometimes, I use them together, first putting on the coconut oil and then the emu oil. Just do not get the coconut oil too close to the eyes because it tends to migrate; however, neither will harm the eyes. If either product gets into the eyes, a little bit of pure water and the dab of a tissue will clear it up.

If you are ever at home during the day, using these nutrients on a clean **face and neck and** the **scalp and eyebrows** will give much beneficial nourishment.

Both of these products penetrate deeply into all layers of the skin. Therefore, another good tip is to **rub this on the neck** before sleeping (or if you are at home in the daytime) **right over the thyroid gland**.

The thyroid is located mid-neck (front) just below the Adam's apple. Coconut oil and emu oil nourish this hardworking gland. Use one oil one week and the other oil the next week.

To read more about coconut oil and its many benefits for the body, access the website of Dr. Mercola, www.mercola.com, and delve into the archives. He is one of many expert sources for information on all things good for the body. One can also go online and read the wealth of information on the thousands of years of history for emu oil and coconut oil, and learn that these incredible oils are **nontoxic, antimicrobial, and anti-inflammatory.** They are the perfect **rub for sore muscles, weary feet, or dry skin** and also **for cuticles on fingers and toes**! MASSAGE with emu for maximum benefit, because it is a thicker consistency while coconut oil is lighter.

WASHING THE FACE, REMOVING MAKEUP

Another fabulous use for ***organic virgin*** coconut oil is for safely removing makeup—including eye makeup—and also washing the face. Yes, replace soap with a product that is nourishing as well as antimicrobial. It also is noncomedogenic (does not clog pores).

Organic virgin coconut oil can additionally be used if there is **acne, rosacea**, or other irritants. It is soothing as opposed to the drying effect of soap.

I buy the thirty-two-ounce size of Omega Nutrition's Organic Virgin Coconut Oil. The "virgin" gives me the purest grade, which is kindest to the pores of the skin. I transfer oil into a three-, four-, or five-ounce jar for easy use and so as not to contaminate the large container.

First, I put some oil onto a very soft tissue and pat/wipe to remove most of my eye makeup. Then I gently pat (no need to rub) the oil all over my face. I use gentle circular motions to loosen the makeup and grime of the day. I like to wear a thin surgical glove. With my eyes closed, I also gently dab the oil over any remaining eye makeup. I then wipe the oil from my glove (it now has makeup on it) with a waiting paper towel. I also have a soft tissue (folded into quarters) waiting, and

I gently wipe my face starting with the oil on my eyes. If there is still mascara left, I put some oil between my thumb and pointer finger and gently rub my lashes in order to remove any mascara. With another tissue, I continue to remove my now-emulsified face makeup. Then I repeat oiling my face and again removing the oil with soft tissues. Twice is usually enough. Sometimes I do this three times.

My skin is left glowing and soft and not dried out from soap and municipal water which, too often, has fluoride and chlorine as well as other contaminants nowadays which are so harmful and irritating. So many pollutants and carcinogens are released into municipal water supplies that it is wise to protect your eyes and skin by using virgin organic coconut oil.

This certainly also *benefits men* since **shaving** can irritate the skin. *This* coconut oil replaces moisture and soothes the skin.

One can also keep the oil in a warm spot near the stove or radiator which will give you warm oil for removing makeup or washing the face. It is delicious! If you like the oil in a more solid state, just keep it in a cool spot. It warms or cools within two to three minutes when kept in a small container.

HAIR REGROWTH and COLOR RESTORATION

The value of emu and coconut oil is already apparent. Being noncomedogenic, the pores are safe. Being nourishing, the pores are replenished.

Many people—especially **men**—have hair follicles that are dormant but not dead. Emu oil has been used for centuries for hair treatment and also for **stopping gray hair from growing** in. I personally used this oil when I noticed some gray hairs starting in my front hairline. I dabbed the emu oil on every night. Lo and behold, after about a month, I noticed that the new hair growing in (behind the gray) was back to my blond. Currently, I alternate and use emu or organic virgin coconut oil. The gray has not returned.

For men and women with dormant follicles, I recommend rubbing the oil all over the scalp every night. Then use a small comb to comb the oil through the hair and to all parts of the scalp. It is not greasy nor will it ruin your pillowcase, but one can always put a second pillowcase over the first one, as well, or a towel. It absorbs into the skin. The history of emu oil can be read online, and it includes being used to **restore hair growth**.

When you wash your hair in the morning, any remnants of the oil will immediately be gone while having nourished the scalp and hair overnight. Again, remember, this is a pure oil with no additives, so it easily absorbs and also easily washes away. As a population, **we are so accustomed to using soap on the face and scalp and having that dried result, so we fail to grasp that a *pure* oil can produce clean skin or hair while *not* deleteriously drying the skin**. Note: If you use hair spray, wash it out before using the oil at bedtime. You want the oil to have total access to the scalp and not get stymied by hair spray.

For nourishing existing hair, both Thunder Ridge Emu Oil and Omega Nutrition Organic Virgin Coconut Oil can be used. Again, use one product this week and the other product next week. Both products definitely enrich the hair and replenish the scalp.

Personal Note: **I am very careful to refer to exactly what products I have used. Success surely depends upon a pure product containing healthy attributes. Other products vary in their ingredients as well as their processing. It took years for me to research and find the products to which I refer. It is also critical that a company can be telephoned and that a customer can speak with a professional representative and get answers to questions.** I also mention this on the "Source List" page because customer service is very important.
SUPPLEMENT: There is one **supplement that has worked for restoring hair color** in some cases. In addition to using the above oils, **PABA** can be used. I used one 500 mg capsule three times daily for four months and then dropped to two capsules daily. In particular, for several dark-haired men, it did indeed reverse their premature graying back to dark hair. There are numerous studies and trials in which PABA has been effective in reversing graying.

Stress can also deplete nutrients, so being sure to get a full complement of balanced **B vitamins** (not megadoses of selected B vitamins but rather nature's balanced protocol) along with PABA (a nonprotein amino acid linked to some B vitamins in helping with certain body functions [including reversing graying hair]) can help the entire body and avoid deficiencies.

Note on nutrient supplement dosing: In taking supplements, I always take Monday and Tuesday as well as the first week of each month off from supplements. I feel that this allows the body some time to clear itself. Additionally, when taking a supplement which is not a vitamin or a mineral nor is it food-based, it is good to stop taking it for three months after being on it for three or four months. This definitely allows the body to eliminate (for example, PABA or herbs) it from one's system (and even assess and observe any positive reactions). Then, when you start over, the body gets a real boost as opposed to just being used to it.

PEYRONIE'S DISEASE (CROOKED OR CURVED PENIS)

Peyronie's disease is where the penis—usually when erect—curves due to plaque that formed and reduced elasticity on one side. Sometimes Peyronie's resolves on its own over time, perhaps due to improved diet and nutrients. **PABA** is one of the nutrient supplements used in many studies that seems to help. Trying the dose mentioned in the previous article can be useful. Additionally, a whole-food diet with foods that are not fractionated can dramatically improve health. Fruits, vegetables, and good fats are so important to body health and supplying nutrients that are critical to overall healthy performance. See all the *Mybyble* articles on good fats, food combining, and nutrients.

COCONUT OR EMU OIL FOR BABIES' AND CHILDREN'S DERRIÈRES BUTTOCK, ANAL, AND RECTAL DISTRESS

Chapped and irritated tushies can cause a lot of crying, ***including for adults***. A pleasant soothing for this discomfort is to dab organic virgin coconut oil or emu oil onto the irritation.

It is also helpful to put the oil onto toilet tissue so that when wiping, one is using something very soft, and this emollient on the tissue transfers to the skin and is soothing and healing. It does not stain one's undergarments. Try both oils, and see which you prefer. I feel that the coconut oil is lighter and seeps into the tissue evenly. You can even prepare some squares of facial tissue (soft facial tissue is often softer than most toilet tissue) or toilet tissue in advance, and have them waiting for when they are needed. The oil stays on the tissue and offers a healing solution.

Emu oil can also be gently introduced into the rectum when one has a situation there. It is easiest to wear thin surgical gloves which keep the fingernails from catching or scratching. This is a wonderful treatment for **hemorrhoids**. I know one lady who used emu oil as she gently pushed a very small hemorrhoid—which was slightly protruding—back into the rectum. She inserted (on a gloved finger) emu oil several times daily for a few days, and the hemorrhoid never protruded again. This is five years ago.

BURN MARKS, AGE SPOTS

Several years ago, I was in my office and proceeded to microwave a cup of water in order to make tea. I opened the microwave door and reached in to get the cup by its handle. I had done this before. Unfortunately, this time the water erupted like a geyser and went all over the top of my hand. It was excruciating.

Someone heard my scream, saw the calamity, and ran to get a bag of ice. A restaurant downstairs sent up more bags of ice over the next several hours. It was that ice—for six hours (after which the pain was gone)—which kept my hand from getting blistered and scarred; however, I wound up with two small freckles (similar to age spots) which were where the burning water first hit the top of my hand. A few years went by when I read that rubbing coconut oil on age spots could help diminish them. I decided to try that for these freckles. Using both Omega Nutrition Organic Coconut Oil and the Virgin Organic Oil (I alternated), I would dab it on every night and numerous times during the day because it sinks right into the skin.

After a month, I noticed that the color of the freckles (or burn spots) was much lighter. Currently, one can barely see them.

SOAP

While emu and coconut oils have their unique place, there are times that we need hand soap and body soap. There are three that I use.

I keep this first bar of soap near my kitchen sink as well as in my bathroom for washing my hands. It is from Omega Nutrition and is the Flax-Orange Handmade Bath Soap. It is handcrafted in small batches using the finest ingredients, including food-grade coconut oil, and leaves the skin smooth (not dried out). The bar is actually filled with tiny flaxseeds, so it is excellent for truly removing dirt and grime (but *not* on the face). *It is* **excellent for men** and for anyone getting really grimy.

The second soap is an unscented liquid, Natural Face & Body Soap from Omega Nutrition. It is superconcentrated and made with natural ingredients. It goes nicely onto a loofah or washcloth in the shower for a total body wash.

My final soap is from Puritan's Pride. It is glycerin soap, is a wonderful value, and comes four bars to a pack. I use it for hand washing as well as in the shower (it is excellent on a loofah or washcloth; I also use it on a toothbrush which is dedicated to washing my toenails with this glycerin soap); however, I only use organic virgin coconut oil on my face. *Personal Note:* I used to use this bar soap on my face. When I developed a bacterial rash on my face (discussed elsewhere in *Mybyble*), I found that the only nonabrasive product was the organic virgin coconut oil. I could gently but thoroughly clean my face without exacerbating the rash.

WASHING HANDS AND BODY: Soap must be in contact with the skin for thirty seconds or more in order to actually clean the skin, and the germs and bacteria *under* the fingernails are the most severe. When your hands are nice and soapy, scrape your nails along the palm of the other hand in order to get soap *under* those nails and remove dirt and germs.

BODY MOVEMENTS TO RELIEVE PAIN, EASE TIRED FEET, FIX HIP, ADJUST JAW, LIFT RIB CAGE, CORRECT SHOULDERS AND POSTURE, ELONGATE SPINE

Whole Body Vibration Unit

So precious is your health! Here are tips for which one might search a lifetime and never find. I consider myself inordinately lucky to have come upon these six movements for the feet, hip, rib cage, jaw, shoulders (posture), and elongating the spine. In fact, it was a miracle . . . actually, six miracles.

One is always looking for ways to relax the body. **Giving the feet a rest can do wonders for the whole body.** You can do this anywhere: at home, the office, at a movie, in the car, on a train or airplane, under the table in a restaurant.

Turn/twist your ankles and feet so the outside of each foot is on the ground and the soles of your feet face each other. You can also do one foot at a time: outer side of foot on the ground and sole facing other foot (which is patiently waiting for its turn). Or you can cross one ankle over the other ankle, again placing the outer sides of the feet on the floor or carpet, which naturally allows the soles of both feet to face outward.

Do this while on the computer or anytime that you are sitting. Since you can do this with your shoes on, there is no special preparation.

This is extremely comforting to one's feet, and this good feeling radiates up through the body.

Personal Note: A brilliant massage therapist in Rotorua, New Zealand, once told me that *massaging—or even resting—the outer side of your heels and midfoot area is critical to good **back health**.* He was massaging my feet and told me that he could feel tightness in the outer side of my heels and the outer middle portion of my feet. He explained that this could indicate current back trouble or future trouble. Thus, whenever my feet are under my desk during a long business day, I slip off my pumps and gently cross my ankles and turn my soles outward, and the relaxed feeling is an immediate pleasure. I also do this in a restaurant (even with my pumps on) or when I am a passenger during a long car drive or on an airplane. **There is joy in knowing that something so simple can offer so much.**

The second maneuver is for the shoulders which also benefits the back, circulation, the lungs, and the arms. It is so easy and logical, and you can move one shoulder at a time or both at the same time. Bring your shoulder forward just a little, then lift it up, and finally bring it as far back as you can. Then just let it drop into place and relax. The shoulder will be positioned into place and maintained by the soft tissue of the back of your shoulder unless, of course, you reach forward for something or bend down in which case the position is displaced. Then just repeat: forward, up, back, and relax.

This is NOT just shoving your shoulders back. This is a maneuver that *lifts* not only the shoulders but the breast, abdomen, and neck.

Sitting at your desk or computer is an excellent time to maintain this shoulders-back position. **You will feel your lungs open up, better breathing, the abdomen firming, and your neck elongating. It is liberating.**

Dr. Mercola wrote about this in his August 25, 2013, e-mail newsletter as he discussed posture as taught by Esther Gokhale (www.mercola.com).

The third maneuver is for elongating the spine. A key factor in alleviating back pain can be elongating the spine. Get down

on all fours, and then extend the right arm and the left leg. The arm points forward with the hand and fingers straight out, your face and eyes are looking at the ground (the neck and chin are *not* craned upward; they are *parallel* to the ground), and the leg has the toes pointed (not flexed). Gently extend the arm forward while stretching the opposite leg backward as you feel your spine elongating. Hold to the count of twenty; then, switch arms and legs. Do twenty. As each movement is executed, hold the stomach in. *Very important*: Do *not* have your eyes looking forward toward your hand, which is a natural tendency. It will throw off your balance. The eyes are looking directly downward. This maintains balance.

I maximize doing this exercise by executing it on a **whole body vibration** unit. It is not one of those $5,000 or $10,000 units but one that I bought from Soloflex for $395. The platform is forty inches long by ten inches wide and five inches high, and the vibrations (when turned on) contract and relax the muscles that you are using for any exercise. This enhances the value of the time that you are spending on the exercise.

I also use my whole body vibration unit when standing up and doing my arm isometrics (see *Mybyble* article on isometrics for the funny bone).

The fourth maneuver is for the hip. One wonders how often certain hip pain is diagnosed as a bone problem needing a hip replacement when, after all, it needs only soft tissue adjustment. It is so easy to determine this simply by doing this maneuver and seeing if it solves the hip pain. Once you have the movement understood, you can do it sitting or standing. Try it for the initial time while standing.

With feet flat on the floor and the big toes slightly pointed toward each other, gently roll both feet *slightly* toward their outer sides while rolling (shifting) the calf muscles inward. In essence, you are trying to pull the back of the legs together without the heels moving. Squeeze the butt while doing this for the added benefit of realigning the pelvis. You will feel—as you rotate the calf muscles inward—the movement go all the way up the leg and behind the buttocks. **This is the key. It is the soft tissue by the hip that needs adjusting. The thigh and**

butt muscles work together for maximum effectiveness. You can also slightly tighten the abdominals for added benefit.

To bring you up-to-date, recently I strained my calf muscle. I performed this exercise and got immediate relief.

You could search extensively (if not for an eternity) and *not* find this information and help. The article mentioned below was the first time that I ever read about it. How nice to share it with you!

Personal Note: How did I come upon this solution? Well, the first question is *why* I needed the solution. I am tall, with long legs. For two days, I was at business meetings where the seats were quite low to the ground. Instead of normal-height chairs, I was (the first day) on a banquet for four hours where **the seat was not deep enough nor high enough** from the ground. By evening, I could feel some **agitation in my left hip**. The second day—this time for a total of six hours—I was at another meeting where I sat on a **sofa that was quite low to the ground**.

By the end of that second day, my back was distressed, and I could feel something in my left hip really bothering me. When I got home, my left hip was in terrible pain, and I thought, *Oh, no. What is with my hip? Am I getting arthritis or something?*

Every night, I read the health e-mail newsletters to which I refer in the *Mybyble* article "Learn". To my absolute astonishment, there was an article in my e-mail on January 11, 2013, from Dr. Mercola referring to this exact topic (sitting, posture, alignment, and exercise/maneuvering). First, I blessed Dr. Mercola. Then I immediately did the exercise and found prompt relief, and by the morning I had no pain. Truly, without that article and the exercise, I would not have been able to sleep that night due to the hip pain and the worry.

The fifth maneuver involves the rib cage. As we age, gravity takes its toll. If we have not been diligent regarding posture (for some this occurs younger than for others), our breastbone area and rib cage sink down. There is a wonderful maneuver to do while sitting or standing. With shoulders back (as described above), gently draw in the stomach and ***then*** lift the rib cage while breathing in. Again: stomach drawn in and then use muscle control and slow deep breathing to raise the rib cage. Feel the lungs open up and the stomach firm and tighten. Now hold the stomach and rib cage in place while, for example, you continue work on your computer, watch television, or read. If you do this often enough, the stomach will naturally assume this position as will the rib cage.

It provides such a good feeling that you will think of it numerous times after first doing it, and thus, it will become habit.

The sixth maneuver is to relax the jaw or to help it recuperate if clicking. Every once in a while, folks will find their jaw clenching or tightening or just feeling peculiar. This can come from stress, excessive talking, or just suddenly moving it the wrong way.

The maneuver is this: Face straight ahead and close your eyes. Slowly move the lower jaw from side to side. Usually, doing this just a few times will reset the jaw into its proper place and ease whatever unhinged it. After doing that maneuver, also gently/slowly move the lower jaw forward and then back to normal position. I find it relaxing.

If you have the unfortunate occurrence of the jaw clicking and also locking when you yawn (in which case you find it painful and difficult to get it moving again), this next procedure is excellent. It was taught to me by a specialist at the Hospital for Joint Diseases in New York City.

Every time you yawn, take the upper side of your hand and hold it under the jaw, causing an isometric effect. You will get the yawn accomplished; however, the jaw will not need to open, and the tension between your hand pressing upward with the jaw trying (but not succeeding) to open downward will create an isometric healing process.

The benefits of isometric exercises are cumulative. The more you do them, the stronger becomes that body part. In this case, the jaw should strengthen and regain its correct position.

If you do not want to hold your hand under the chin, you can also lower the chin to press against the neck every time you yawn. Again, the neck pressing into the chin will prevent an openmouthed yawn and will offer that isometric tension for healing.

Personal Note: It is humorous how I came to need help with my jaw. It started when I was nine years old. I used to run to the door to great my Dad when he came home from business every night. This one night, I ran, jumped into his arms, and as he was turning his head to kiss me, I turned my head too quickly and whacked my jaw into his jaw, and I dislocated my jaw.

He immediately called an orthopedic surgeon whom we knew (the brilliant, kind, and incomparable Dr. Irving Glick) who said to bring me right to his office. He had his miniature poodle there to cuddle with me and take my attention away from my jaw while he quietly reassured me and placed his fingers in my mouth. Suddenly, he gave a pull, and voilà, my jaw was set back into place.

Fast forward thirty years, and I am reclined ninety degrees on my home gymnasium after a hard day's work. I suddenly needed to yawn and opened to give a really wide, exhausted yawn, and *pop*—something clicked, and my jaw, while not dislocated, was out of place. Dr. Glick was sadly no longer alive, and I searched high and low for someone who would stick his fingers in my mouth, pull, and reset the jaw.

I can tell you how many quacks I consulted with: three! Not one of them understood what I needed, and one had the audacity to tell me that I had arthritis and should see his physical therapist twice a week forevermore. You get the picture. I would be just another cash cow.

By the way, I heard this same doctor (when I was waiting in an adjoining examining room) tell an eighty-eight-year-old gentleman that the **black-and-blue spots on his hands** and arms were from age and needed to be treated (again by his therapist) with a laser for about twelve months. This, of course, was hogwash. I caught up with this elderly man outside and told him that **the spots were caused by lack of bioflavonoids** (which are found in the pith [the white substance just under the skin] of citrus fruits). I assured him that it was nutrients he needed and not a laser. He immediately agreed with me and said, "That doc is a quack, in my opinion," and told me that despite his age, he was excellent on a computer and asked if I could e-mail him what he should buy. We exchanged addresses; I did e-mail the information to him, and over several months, he let me know about his progress. He did listen to me, and he did get rid of all the black-and-blue spots. Note that those spots were *not* bruises. Bruises would need different treatment (whole vitamin C, vitamin K2, calcium, and magnesium; see *Mybyble* article on "Heart Palpitations," which discusses these nutrients) while *his spots* were a symptom of his nutrient deficiency (whole vitamin C and bioflavonoids).

Back to my jaw dilemma: At that time, I had recently been a junior trustee at the Hospital for Joint Diseases (I had to resign due to my extensive business travel; I was never in New York for the meetings), so I called the head of the hospital and explained my predicament, and he immediately told me that he would set up an appointment for me with their specialist in the jaw area. It was this doctor who taught me to press my hand to my jaw (or press my jaw to my neck) and that the jaw would strengthen and be corrected quickly. He was right! Within five days my jaw was perfect.

Honestly, though, to this day I do not open wide to yawn. I always hold my hand under my jaw as a preventive.

ELONGATE THE SPINE WHILE SITTING

Sitting can be so detrimental to back health. People forget to keep their shoulders back (which raises the chest and expands the lungs and keeps the head well-positioned and not drooping) and maintain a firm stomach.

Of great benefit is having a rolled towel or a rolled pillow behind you in the lumbar region (lower spine) in order to keep your back from crunching into the chair. Instead, this accessory elongates the spine and allows the discs to rehydrate and keeps nerves from pinching. It supports the lumbar region and promotes better sitting posture. Exactly what size pillow or rolled towel is used depends upon the chair shape. Try a few until you are ready to say "Ahhhhh!"

LENGTHEN/STRENGTHEN THE NECK

This is **so easy** and able to be used anywhere in order to **enhance your appearance**. There is nothing worse than to see someone schlumping along on the sidewalk or sitting and looking like a schlump because the head is not held erect. To give yourself that air of importance (while enhancing your own health), *pretend that you are a puppet, and the top of your head has strings attached to it which are being pulled up by the puppeteer.*

Feel those strings pulling **the top of your head** *up.* Feel your neck straighten and your chin firm up. **Look in the mirror and see the difference.**

FIRM THE CHIN

Hold the top of the **tongue to the roof of the mouth. Look in the mirror,** and see the difference when your chin is held the usual way versus being taut when the tongue firms it up from this roof-top position. Once you start holding the tongue to the roof of the mouth, it becomes a healthy habit.

WRINKLES, EXPRESSIONS
MIRROR, MIRROR ON THE WALL

It may be the shock of your life if you look into a mirror and start talking to yourself, laughing, grimacing, and doing whatever you normally do when speaking with another person. Just wait until you see the way your face changes from that smooth facade which you see in the mirror when doing makeup or shaving—when your face is still and you are not animated.

Difficult as this may be, this is a lesson in facial movement and habit. You can teach yourself *out* of making those faces. At home (or in your office if you have privacy), place a mirror near your telephone. Watch your face while you speak with people. You can catch those grimaces and other movements and train yourself to correct them. Then when you are with people, it will be in the back of your mind *not* to make those faces.

FROWNING

Train yourself <u>out</u> of frowning. If you notice that you are developing frown lines, you can work at training yourself to stop frowning. Here is a good tip: Watch other people's faces! See their wrinkles and frown marks, and you will surely not do it!

Frowning—for many people—becomes a habit, especially when one is thinking while, for example, washing hands or dishes or during other concentrated tasks. One way to refocus your concentration is to close your eyes. Then you are simply washing hands or dishes.

CLENCH YOUR FIST TO REMEMBER

Clenching your fist may temporarily change the way your brain functions in a way that boosts memory. Those who clenched a ball in their right hand before memorization and in their left hand before recall boosted their memory scores by 15 percent compared to a control group. This memory trick works, because making a fist can increase activity in the brain on the opposite side (so if you clench your right fist, activity in the left brain hemisphere increases).

IF YOU ARE TALL, DON'T SHRINK

It is no joke. For taller folks, we are always bending down to things: kitchen sinks, bathroom sinks, tables, and even to shorter people. Our shoulders sag and, over the years, so does the spine. It collapses.

Household fixtures, such as sinks, are installed at a height that is considered standard and *is* standard for what was *once* the average person's height. This has never been revised. Over the years, this takes a toll on one's posture and health.

Go ahead. Go to your kitchen or bathroom sink, and wash your hands. Now tell me that you see how you let your shoulders drop and your arms lower. In fact, the shoulders should be kept **rolled back** (see *Mybyble* article "Body Movements . . . Correct Shoulders and Posture") which will keep the **upper arms close** to the body and basically just your lower arms and hands functioning (whether in the sink, on the computer, or in doing other tasks). It quickly becomes second nature, though, and then you are always aware of this when you tend to slouch, and you correct it promptly.

Those rolled-back shoulders will be a blessing for your body as the years progress.

Remember when you are doing tasks to keep yourself erect—even when washing dishes or peeling an apple over the garbage can. Keep those shoulders rolled back, bend from the waist as opposed to dropping the shoulders and slouching, and sit ***up!***

Personal Note: Please enjoy a good laugh on me! While I was proofreading this manuscript and changing wording here and there, I could not help but adjust my sitting posture and get my shoulders up every time I read one of my shoulder and/or posture articles. I would be so engrossed with my work that I suddenly realized that I was not following my own advice. So, I put a tiny sticky-note on the edge of my computer monitor as a constant reminder to *sit up*!

SCOLIOSIS: ONE SHOULDER LOWER THAN THE OTHER

This condition can be from childhood or develop later in life. A bad fall can cause a maladjustment, and **one day you look in the mirror** when you are undressed, and you see that **one shoulder is lower than the other**. This second scenario happened to me. If neglected, this imbalance will get worse.

I suffered a severe fall overseas, where my high heel slid into a sidewalk crack, and I fell over backward. Aside from pulling my back, the muscles from my knee to my groin in my right leg were terribly injured. It took three months to walk without crutches.

A few months went by, and I started noticing that (sometimes) if I suddenly turned my head right or left, I got *a sharp jolt of pain that shot up from my shoulder into my ear*. It brought tears to my eyes. No one could explain it.

Sometime after that, I was on business overseas, came out of the shower, and suddenly saw myself in the mirror. It was seeing myself outside of my normal home bathroom (where one does not pay so much attention) that caught my eye. My right shoulder was slightly lower than my left. I was in shock.

Slowly, over several days, I mentally pieced together the lowered shoulder and the jolts of pain in my neck when sometimes turning my head swiftly. I connected all this to that fall. Certainly, I had friends with scoliosis; however, they had this from childhood, but I knew about that symptom of the lower shoulder.

When I returned home, I started researching scoliosis. After much reading, I had the tremendous pleasure of finding the CLEAR Scoliosis Institute (www.clear-institute.org). CLEAR stands for Chiropractic Leadership, Educational Advancement, and Research. It is a nonprofit organization dedicated to improving scoliosis treatment without surgery or bracing and was started by the incomparable Dr. Dennis Woggon, founder and CEO. In May 2010, I wrote to his dedicated son Dr. Josh Woggon, Director of Research: "My involvement in real health care is what makes me so grateful for YOU because you are the Lone Ranger in scoliosis and related conditions! I do not imagine that anyone else has accomplished what you have."

One can sign up to receive e-mails which are very informative. CLEAR also trains chiropractic doctors who practice all over the world and provide CLEAR treatment. I located one a few hours from my home and met with the doctor who treats patients of all ages. I learned about the treatment that focuses on correcting the curve and, hence, the lower shoulder. This is where I learned more about whole body vibration units (see in *Mybyble*) and doing the arm isometrics while on the unit. See *Mybyble* article "Funny Bone and Isometrics", because isometrics are very helpful in correcting the curve and easing symptoms (the isometrics got rid of those jolts in my neck [from shoulder to ear]). As the *Mybyble* article advises, as you do the isometrics, watch yourself (undressed) in the mirror—front, sides, and back—and you will see the skin and muscle behind your armpit raise up on the side of the body that needs to raise up, the side with the lowered shoulder.

In reference to the previous article ("If You Are Tall, Don't Shrink") which mentions the height of many homes' fixed appliances, note that people who favor their dominant arm (if right-handed, they lower the right shoulder in order to do more with the right hand in the sink, for example; if writing, the shoulder of the dominant arm tends to dip; if handing something to someone, you reach out with your dominant hand and drop the shoulder) will, later in life, find that shoulder placement deteriorated along with a possible curve in the back. It is SO important to maintain good posture at all times. Those rolled-back shoulders will provide many blessings in later years.

FOOD COMBINING
Weight, Gas, Bloating, Digestive Problems

Do **not ever mix fruits and vegetables** (except for apples). They require different digestive enzymes and taken together throw the stomach into a tizzy.

Do **not eat potatoes with meat**. The stomach cannot digest them together. Proteins do not combine with starches. Potatoes **alone** are a wonderful entrée. If you dine in a restaurant and you are served meat with potatoes (or any other improperly combined foods), take home the potatoes! Doggie bags are de rigueur in the fight for a safe diet. Your health is more important that worrying about carrying a doggie bag.

Do **not eat fruit after a meal**. It sits on top of the food and rots everything in the stomach. It causes the process of digestion to slow horrendously (see article "Digestion/Indigestion"). When **you improperly combine foods, they putrefy in the stomach. Everything rots, and you get no nutrients from what you just ate!**

Fruit should be eaten alone—and on an empty stomach—in the morning with a two—hour, **or more**, wait before eating other food. If you eat melon, it should be eaten alone. It digests the most quickly, and if eaten with other fruit, there is a digestive problem. Never combine melon with other food groups.

You ask, "What do you mean? How can this be true?" Well, it is (!), and **the extended life span causes many more burdens on the human body and its systems**. Mistreatment of the body accumulates, and indigestion, acid reflux, constipation, rashes, and excess weight are only a few of the many *symptoms* of poor digestion due to improper food combining. I ask *you*: Do you mix any of the food groups mentioned above? If yes, are you ever in for digestive trouble**s**!

Harvey and Marilyn Diamond's book *Fit for Life* provided the first information that I ever read on food combining. One can also Bing or Google "Food combining rules" and get a wealth of health information. (See *Mybyble* article "Digestion/Indigestion" tips.)

People complain of stomach and digestion problems all the time. One of the easiest ways toward weight loss, no bloating, no gas, and relieving digestive and other health issues is through proper food combining. Improper food combining creates a toxic atmosphere in the stomach that makes blood more acidic which allows yeast, viruses, infections, parasites, cancer cells, and other virulent results to develop because undigested food is putrefying.

Now you have a better understanding of easy corrections that can be made to your eating habits in order to put your tummy in order. Smile and think of me as your tummy thanks *you*. **Years from now you *will* thank *Mybyble* for this!**

WEIGHT LOSS, WEIGHT CONTROL, DIET
The Body Needs Good Fats, WHOLE Foods, and NOT Fractionated Foods

This is a critical issue to most everyone. Since food combining was just addressed, it is important to mention individually the topic of weight.

First, proper food combining will enhance weight control. When a person stops eating food groups which cannot be digested when eaten together in one meal, digestion will be released from the burden of a tizzy in the stomach due to putrefying meals, one will consume less food *because* properly eaten food will now be digested and provide nutrition thus relieving/preventing hunger pangs, and the body will finally start receiving nutrients from properly digested food. This will indeed enhance weight control, and it is so easy. **No dieting**. Just eat meals of individual food groups. See the results over a one-month time.

Secondly, as an alternative approach, when one decides to diet, an easy way to start is to eat what you normally do but <u>only eat *half* of what is on the plate</u>. Remember that ***it takes twenty minutes for the stomach to let the brain know that it is full.*** You need to ***eat slowly,*** and CHEW every mouthful at least twenty times. Saliva and chewing will get the digestive juices flowing and awaiting the arrival of well-chewed food to the stomach.

After a couple of weeks, one will develop the habit of chewing (which rewards you with slower eating and waiting for the stomach to tell the brain that it is *full*) and portion control. If you are in a restaurant, doggie bags tote home the remaining food. You are not deprived of favorite foods. You are just eating less of the same foods.

The third suggestion will find a receptive audience in both those having moderate trouble avoiding unhealthy foods as well as **binge eaters**. We know that once food is swallowed, any satisfaction from gustation is past. Therefore, whether the food is swallowed or expectorated has no effect on the pleasure from chewing it and sensing the satisfaction. Yes, I said: Spit it out. Contrary to the dangers of purposely throwing up which should *never* be done, expectorating will not harm the body but will satisfy the need for a taste. There is, after all, no satisfaction from a swallow.

"Taste and spit" in this regard is **similar to wine tasting**, where one tastes a number of wines and expectorates. One *still* gets the full flavor and pleasure without getting drunk. So, spit out unnecessary food and do not get sick or fat!

In the privacy of one's home or office, the intense need for cake or any food (such as the dangerous fried foods) can be satisfied with *briefly* chewing it and then expectorating right into the garbage can or a small plastic bag. Have another bite. Just do not swallow it. This will slowly develop a new thought process which is: Having just a small bite (and swallowing it) is just as satisfying as uncontrolled eating. Anything after the first swallowed mouthful really offers no additional pleasure because, in fact, **your memory of a taste can be sufficiently satisfying** as opposed to eating yourself sick.

May I add a thought: Please do not comment "Yuck!". There are so many issues related to eating, and this third suggestion can help some folks satisfy certain cravings for not-so-healthy foods and, more importantly, also aid others who seriously overeat and need help developing an exit path.

The fourth comment is for everyone and will enhance the health of the entire body as well as weight control. *The body needs good fats*—not trans fats, not hydrogenated. Good fats are, for example, cultured butter (preferably from pastured cows); goat milk; organic coconut oil; grass-fed organic beef, venison, buffalo, pork; cage-free organic chicken; organic eggs from cage-free chickens; nonprocessed cheese. The list goes on. *The body would starve without proper fats which are critical in nourishing the brain, the nerves, the skin, almost all other organs, and much more. When someone lacks these fats, they wither.* Skin and hair show all the symptoms of this deficiency with dryness and poor general condition. **When these external symptoms appear, one knows that there are problems internally. Mental issues can develop from a deficiency of good fats.**

Fats are also necessary for the body to absorb fat-soluble vitamins, reduce inflammation, and prevent disease. Remember that there are nutrients in vegetables and fruits which are fat soluble. Therefore, anyone eating a low-fat or no-fat diet will fail to absorb these vital nutrients.

The body also needs <u>whole</u> foods. It cannot thrive on **fractionated, low-fat, no-fat**, et al. In other words, when a food is separated from its natural, integral ingredients, the stomach cannot recognize it. An altered food becomes nonsupportive of total health and is indigestible. That is why people on these diets always feel hungry or malnourished. They are consuming incomplete items which are sold as food, and this leaves the body searching for sustenance.

Learn to **eat whole foods** in moderation. *The stomach will size itself to accommodate what you put into it.* As you consume portions that support a healthy weight for your size, the stomach will become satisfied with those portions. Learn the names of producers of organic, whole-food products so that when you shop, you can gravitate to those items.

TIPS FOR BURNING CALORIES: Going for a **walk after dinner** is one of the best things you can do for your weight. Why? Because **you will use up some of your dinner calories** that **would otherwise get stored as fat** while one sleeps. Many folks have lost a lot of weight by going for a walk before bedtime. I highly recommend it. And if you swing those arms over the head while walking, you will burn more calories faster.

The second-best time for walking to burn fat is **before** breakfast, because if you wait until you give your body some fuel (food), it will use that instead of your fat stores for energy. In the morning, you want to burn stored fat as opposed to newly ingested food.

DRINK WARM WATER

Start the day with a cup of warm water. It hydrates the body, cleanses and tones the digestive system, and gets peristalsis going. Many enjoy some fresh lemon and/or raw honey in the hot water. It is also beneficial to drink some pure warm water before bedtime. It flushes fats out of the stomach, reduces the concentration of bile which can awaken people to urinate, and can also provide hydration which leads to better sleep. I drink warm water all day.

PROBIOTICS FOR GUMS AND PERIODONTAL DISEASE 'PULLING' FOR GUM HEALTH

In September 2013 I received unique product information from a medical news outlet about a probiotic mint lozenge. While there are probiotics for the gut (see next article), to see one that focuses on the gums is rare. All probiotics are not the same. The benefits are strain specific. Prodentis was designed to help balance the oral environment and thus provide a natural defense against unhealthy teeth and gums, plaque, and bad breath. GUM PerioBalance begins working with the very first lozenge to help build the level of good bacteria (Prodentis) in the mouth, and positive changes in gum and oral health were viewed during the first twenty-eight days of use (in clinical trials of which, currently, there have been more than twenty-five).

In one study, it was shown that *Lactobacillus reuteri* Prodentis acts synergistically with standard treatment (scaling and root planing [SRP]) to significantly reduce probing pocket depth (PPD) and clinical attachment level (CAL) which are the two most important parameters in assessing the severity of periodontitis. Furthermore, *L. reuteri* Prodentis reveals—as the first probiotic ever—significant reductions of three different pathogens in patients with chronic periodontitis. The study also confirms the anti-inflammatory effects of *L. reuteri* Prodentis on gum inflammation (gingivitis).

Chronic periodontitis occurs in up to 40 percent of the adult population. The standard treatment aims at removing plaque in the dental pockets to reduce the periodontal pathogens and thereby prevent disease progression. The result showed that a combination of *L. reuteri* Prodentis and SRP was significantly better than all other modalities in reducing gingivitis and plaque. Moreover, *L. reuteri* Prodentis, either alone or following SRP, significantly reduced several pathogens by up to 90 percent as compared to the treatments that did not include *L. reuteri* Prodentis.

This short-term study advises that *L. reuteri* Prodentis by itself has a powerful effect on the pathogens of periodontitis, and the combination of *L. reuteri* Prodentis and SRP synergistically improves both PPD and CAL. The results strengthen the *L. reuteri* Prodentis position as a treatment option for patients with periodontal disease. View http://periobalance.com for company information and where to buy. The parent is a Swedish company, BioGaia.

Personal Note: I immediately decided to try this due to two areas of my gums that were tender when being flossed. I also put a gentleman who had periodontal issues on this regimen. Within thirty days, the tenderness in my gums was hugely diminished, and by forty days, it was gone. With the gentleman having issues, the inflammation and bleeding when he brushed were gone in forty days.

Second Personal Note: Combining GUM PerioBalance—which is a <u>strain-specific</u> probiotic for the mouth—with Good-Gums (see article "GOOD-GUMS FOR HEALTHY BRUSHING OF TEETH"), one can significantly improve mouth health. Here are some tips: **First,** before bed, floss and brush (with Good-Gums) the teeth. **Then** pop the mint lozenge GUM PerioBalance into the mouth. You want to *slowly* keep it dissolving for at least ten minutes in order to flood the gums with the healing juices from the lozenge. Read something you enjoy for those few minutes, and each time that your saliva produces some mint "juice", swoosh it through your teeth, BUT do a procedure called **PULLING.**

This is one of the greatest tips! Tilt your head forward and direct the mint juice to and through six areas: top left, top front, top right, lower right, lower middle, and lower left. Repeat several times. **PULL** the saliva juice **through** the teeth. This is different than just swooshing it around. PULLING (and one should **absolutely do this with Good-Gums** in order to get its healing nutrients really working on the teeth and gums) **draws out tiny pieces still there, removes bacteria, and soothes gums.**

PULLING comes from an old practice called Oil Pulling which nowadays can be done using Omega Nutrition Organic Virgin Coconut Oil. Its antimicrobial power is very helpful with gums which, as one *pulls* the oil through the teeth, "pulls out" bacteria, viruses, fungi, and other debris. Spit out at end. Dr. Mercola has written about this. **Pulling is both preventive and therapeutic. In a therapeutic situation, the longer one pulls with any of these solutions (Good-Gums, GUM PerioBalance, Celtic sea salt water, organic virgin coconut oil) the better!** Since these products are natural and food based, there is no harm if something is swallowed. See "Source List" for purchasing.

Going back to the mint lozenge, doing this **at bedtime allows the healing properties to remain in the gums and on the teeth for the whole night**. One cannot imagine (until doing this) the benefits to the gums and teeth. Yes, one can definitely swallow the mint juices, but the saliva-liquefied Good-Gums juice should be spit out after pulling or swooshing. And no, **one does not need to do both procedures**. If you just want to use Good-Gums for brushing and swooshing, the rewards are significant as is.

Secondly, use Celtic sea salt water to swoosh or do pulling all during the day. See article "Salt Water". I keep a big china mug premade in order to swoosh after any meal or snack.

PROBIOTICS
Getting Rid of that Paunch and Some Inches

I researched for a long time before finding the Mt. Capra products. Since I am a great believer in goat milk (see next article), I was very happy to find Mt. Capra and Caprobiotics Plus+. It is all natural, no chemicals, no preservatives, and **is the only brand of probiotics cultured in goat milk**. It is sourced from free-range goats and is gluten-and GMO-free. There are several Mt. Capra choices. I like Caprobiotics Plus+ because it delivers the maximum potency in just one or two capsules. Some days I take one; other days I take two.

It contains over thirty billion beneficial bacteria per two-capsule serving, with ten synergistic strains of live and active cultures in each capsule. This Goat Milk Plus+ Blend includes prebiotics. *Compare this to other product labels*. I find that others fall short.

For years I pooh-poohed probiotics. I thought, *Who needs that!* Fairly recently—about fifteen months ago—I received some research which goaded me into trying them. In particular, it focused on putting the intestinal tract in good order, **good health emanating from a healthy gut**, getting rid of waste, and flattening the tummy. **Probiotics are living, healthy bacteria which deliver health benefits to the gastrointestinal tract** when correctly ingested. They replenish intestinal microflora which helps the body digest and absorb food as well as **fight off many illnesses and disease**. After a few weeks, I was amazed to find that the small puffiness of my tummy had disappeared. I decided that what I saw on the outside of my body indicated that good things were going on inside.

GOAT'S MILK
Cow's Milk Is Meant for Baby Cows

The sweetest, smoothest, nutritious milk is goat milk. In many parts of the world, it is drunk much more than in the United States.

Why goat milk? Do you ever notice how you keep trying to clear your throat after ice cream, a glass of milk, or having tea or coffee with milk or cream from cows? That is the clogging effect. Many people have sensitivities to cow's milk which ***is mucus forming***. Also, the fat globules in goat's milk are one-ninth the size of those in cow's milk which is another possible reason that it does not produce irritation in the gut.

Goat's milk is closer to human mother's milk than to cow's milk. Because it has a chemical makeup that is much closer to human milk, it is easier to digest and assimilate in the human body. It also benefits in weight control: It **has less fat** but maintains high levels of proteins and amino acids as well as calcium, selenium, and the amino acid tryptophan. It **is nutrient dense**.

One cannot freeze and then successfully defrost cow's milk; however, I can freeze small amounts of goat milk, defrost it, and use it. To view the purity of goat milk, pour all the milk out of a bottle. The goat milk bottle is clean; there are no specks all over it.

In New York, I buy Oak Knoll Goats' Milk. I also enjoy it in chocolate and half-and-half cream. The first time that I tasted this milk, I exclaimed, "Mmmmm . . . this is the sweetest, most perfect milk! *This* is how milk should taste." I still think this when I have a glass or two of milk each day. Additionally, if I stir in a scoop of Jay Robb Chocolate Whey Protein and let it sit for fifteen minutes, it becomes a **luscious, frothy chocolate shake**. If I then put the glass in the freezer for about an hour, I have the most delicious chocolate frosted. The chocolate whey totally assimilates into the goat milk and gives me added protein to that already provided by the goat milk.

This goat milk is free of antibiotics and hormones. No pesticides are used on their non-GMO crops where the goats graze. Now you are informed as to what to look for on labels of the milk you buy as well as reasons to buy goat milk.

Goats are one of the smallest domesticated ruminants that have served mankind earlier and longer than cattle and sheep.

HUM FOR HEALTHY VOCAL CORDS

The only surefire remedy for a strained voice is humming. Whispering or speaking in a pitch other than your normal one is <u>*not*</u> good. It strains the voice further. It is unnatural.

If you have overused your voice or yelled, hum! It relieves the throat by vibrating the vocal cords and relaxing them. The sooner that one hums following an argument or a lengthy speech, the better for one's vocal cords. Humming soothes them. Choose a few songs that—for you—are hummable. You can also hum scales.

Also, if your throat has been overused, gargle with George's Always Active® Aloe Vera. It soothes (and can also be swallowed). One can also suck on Thayers Slippery Elm Lozenges which have provided relief since 1847. Made from the inner bark of the Slippery Elm tree (*Ulmus fulva*), these dependable demulcents soothe the tissues of the mouth and throat and ease the voice without the dulling effects of menthol.

In order to strengthen your voice, **hum for ten minutes daily**. Hum while walking, dressing, blowing hair dry, driving the car, or washing dishes . . . even on the toilet.

As one ages, humming can keep vocal cords strong, resilient, and tuneful. Humming can maintain a firm and resonant voice. It is also never too late to start humming!

Personal Note: How did I learn this? I was in my twenties and had given a speech. After my presentation, a beautiful woman introduced herself to me. She was the renowned speech coach/teacher Dorothy Sarnoff (formerly, opera singer and Broadway actress). She complimented my speech and then gave me a tip to last my lifetime (which *Mybyble* gives to you): "Hum to keep your vocal cords healthy." We then had a wonderful conversation about humming and all the people (singers, actors, and business leaders) taught to hum by the lovely and accomplished Dorothy Sarnoff.

FLASHLIGHT USES

Nighttime: One always wants to sleep in total darkness in order to get the best and deepest sleep. Should you need to go to the bathroom, you do not want to turn on bright lights which will disturb your ability to fall back to sleep. Keep a small flashlight near the bed, and let it illumine your path to the bathroom. These tiny LED flashlights are quite powerful. They are now the size of a lipstick or pen, so they take up no room.

In a purse or a briefcase: Always carry a miniflashlight. If you drop something between the seats in the car (or anywhere else), it is wonderful to have that bright light finding what is missing. **And, one never knows what a day might bring:**

Personal Note: **September 11, 2001**, started out as a beautiful, sunny morning until Manhattan was attacked. My office was on Wall Street and just several blocks east of the World Trade Towers. I stayed there all day and then went (walking through ankle-deep ashes in a silent downtown, except for sirens in the distance) to The Regent Hotel on Wall Street which was using a generator for power. The ballroom was thrown open so that police and firemen could be bused over from the burning Towers and get food and water and sit down for a while. I helped serve those men (whose uniforms were shredded from the jagged pieces of steel, and gloves were torn and burned, while their faces were etched in pain and grime) and get them supplies (such as aspirin) when possible. The story is much longer than this; however, later when the hotel general manager gave me the key to my accommodation and I went upstairs (climbing twelve flights of stairs with my calves and front of legs in agony from climbing up and down over 200 flights of stairs that horrific day), I entered the hallway which was in total darkness. In all my life, I had never been in a situation where I could not see my hand in front of my face!

The general manager had given me a big, fat banquet candle (he was not providing candles to other guests, but he knew me and took pity on me) and matches and pleaded with me, "Please, please, Mrs. Steiner, please do not burn down my hotel."

Well, when I reached that pitch darkness and was going to light the candle, I suddenly remembered that I had a tiny flashlight in my purse. When I flew Lufthansa, it was one of the gifts in the travel bag, and I always left it in my purse. I fished around in my bag in the dark and found the little light. All that I had to do was squeeze it to provide light.

That was my lesson for life: keep a miniflashlight with you at all times. I also wrote to the chairman of Lufthansa. I asked him, "Do you ever wonder if any of the gifts that you give out are useful? Well, I can tell you that my Lufthansa light lit my way on that horrific night in Manhattan." He was delighted to receive my letter and shared it with the president of Lufthansa USA as well as with many other executives. They also sent me the most magnificent huge basket of Christmas cookies, chocolates, and cakes.

SHORT-TERM MEMORY LOSS

At some point in life, many develop short-term memory loss. **To remember what just slipped your mind, invert your body either by:**

- going on a slant board (lying with head to ground and feet upward);
- standing on your head (there are cushioned units available in exercise-equipment stores to facilitate standing on one's head; the shoulders are cushioned while there is a hole for the head to lower through but not touch the ground);
- lying on a bed facing the headboard, putting stockinged feet up on the back wall;
- or even lying down on the carpet and putting the legs up onto a chair or bed (place a pillow or fluffy towel under your head to cushion it; in this position on the carpet or floor, one can further hasten blood flow to the head by raising the pelvis; keep your arms flat on the floor or carpet [palms down] and raise pelvis).

What slipped your mind will usually come back within minutes, if not moments. The flow of nourishing blood to the brain will also relax you and clarify a lot of other thoughts.

Personal Note: I find that reclining almost upside down (ninety degrees on my West Bend gymnasium [now the company is called Total Gym]) sends nourishing blood to the brain as well as to the face and improves skin tone. It also puts the body organs into their proper place when gravity has sucked them downward. This is a big help for digestion. The rare times that I feel that my digestion needs tweaking, I lie upside down after a meal, and within minutes, my stomach feels better (see next article).

HANG UPSIDE DOWN OR, AT LEAST, PARTIALLY INVERTED
Back Issues, Digestion, Circulation, Brain and Eye Nourishment, Skin

One of the most wonderful treats/treatments to give oneself is to invert the body. **You feel everything fall into proper alignment as you undo the deleterious effects of gravity.**

I used to get intense lower backache, not pain, but stiffening, locking, and various quirks; not all at once, but at different times. Aside from finding out that I was short of vitamin D3 (see following article, "Back Problems")—which took care of much of the problem—**I learned that the lower back is a center for all nerve impulses; if one is under great strain, it can manifest itself in lower-back problems where there is a network of nerves.**

Well, for years I had a home gymnasium that went unused because I never had enough time. There is a five-foot laddered stand at one end with nine levels to which one can attach a leather board (that also slides up and down for exercising). So if lying inverted, one's head is at the end of a board near the ground while one's feet are up near the top or wherever it is comfortable (usually hooking the toes under a bar at the top in order to stretch out the body; I always wrap Turkish towels around these bars in order to cushion my legs and toes). One can adjust how high the board goes (but it is always short of ninety degrees), and I recommend starting where the body is on a gentle slant and, day by day, increasing the height (of where the board attaches to the ladder).

Going back to my comment that I had this gymnasium sitting unused: In agony one evening and having read somewhere of the benefits of inversion, I swung myself onto the board, hooking my toes under an upper rung, and gingerly I lowered myself backward. I reached my arms behind my head and placed my hands against a wall about six inches behind my head, and oh! the relief! Relaxation flooded over my body.

I knew to only do this for five minutes the first time. A few hours later I extended it, and after a few days, I stayed for twenty minutes which I try to continue to this day. If I cannot do a full twenty minutes, I try to do five-minute segments at different times of the day.

Any minutes are better than none; however, great benefits are derived from a longer time.
I do eye, neck, and arm exercises while there as well as deep breathing. I play music that I enjoy and time my session according to how many songs get played.

One can get a bit stiff sometimes as lymph glands empty (so to speak). You can always sit up and readjust. When you sit up, maintain good posture: chest out, shoulders back. This will naturally tighten your abdomen and stomach. **Take a deep breath before continuing or getting up.** Always *ease* out of an exercise or position so that the body is not strained.

As I earlier wrote, I wrap a nice fluffy towel around the rung where I hook my toes and put a plumped sheet or towel under my knees. **IMPORTANT:** Remember to **keep the back flat against whatever you are lying on**. There is a tendency for *the lower back* to arch a bit. DO NOT DO THAT! You want to **keep the back and lower back flat into the board** or support item in order to prevent straining it.

See article "Breathing, Arm Exercises, and Neck Exercises" for what I do to pass the time on the slanted board.

Of course, everyone does not have a gym. One can purchase slant pads at exercise equipment stores or, sometimes, in those departments at Kmart and similar stores.

One can also fashion one's own board by going to a lumberyard and using some imagination. Then, to cushion one's back, use a pad that one would place on a chaise lounge.

You can get some benefit from inversion by lying on your back on the floor (carpeted or cushioned with towels or similar) and putting your legs up on a bed. Enhance this by keeping arms flat next to the body (palms down) and raising the pelvis which stretches out the back, tightens the stomach, and gets blood flow to the head more quickly.

Standing on the head is also good, although I do not do this. There is a padded shoulder armrest that one can utilize which has a hole for the head to go through but <u>not</u> touch the ground while the padding supports the shoulders. Exercise equipment stores sell this.

Digestion: Reclining at a ninety-degree angle (or even less) is also supportive of digestion as well as **nourished skin, eyes, and brain**. By enhancing the blood flow to the upper parts of the body, we gain health benefits while also reaping the benefits of taking back what gravity pulls down.

Every once in a while, my stomach does not digest a lunch or dinner well. Stress, of course. I swing onto my gymnasium board, slowly recline backward, and can immediately feel my organs relaxing into place. After a couple of minutes or longer, my stomach feels better as **digestive juices** react to this easing position.

Footnote: The famous, irreplaceable designer Pauline Trigère was fabulous until her passing in 2002 (born 1908 or 1909 depending upon what biography one reads). In an article at that time, I recall a marvelous comment attributing benefitting her looks, brains, and energy to standing on her head every morning in order "to bathe the brain". "Better than a facial," the wonderful Ms. Trigère commented. It was also written that she and her boyfriend enjoyed a good relationship. He was a younger man by ten years, and they were together since 1952. She looked so stunning and refused to reveal her age until she gave herself a 90th birthday party in 1998 where her age on the invitation was printed—in keeping with her vibrant wit—upsidedown! So, yes!, stand on *your* head or invert the body for benefitting your health while upsidedown.

BACK DISCOMFORT

At one time I had on-and-off back discomfort (especially stiffness upon arising in the morning or getting up from a seat in the theater or the movies). In one health newsletter ("Second Opinion," at that time written by Dr. Douglass), the medical doctor mentioned that some people need more vitamin D3 than others and that chronic back pain may indicate such a need. (See *Mybyble* article "Learn" where Dr. William Campbell Douglass is mentioned.)

I immediately upped my intake to 800 IUs daily (half in the morning, half in the evening). It worked! No more stiffness or pain after a few weeks! Dr. Douglass was the first person that I knew of who wrote about the need for vitamin D3 for lower-back pain. Many articles and much research followed, including what the dosage should be.

Currently, I take 1,000 IUs five times daily (with two days off per week and one week off per month) as current research shows our bodies' needs for D3. I also receive e-mails from the Vitamin D Council (info@vitamindcouncil.org) (www.vitamindcouncil.org). One should do a simple blood test regarding vitamin D levels. Information is available from both the Vitamin D Council and www.mercola.com.

Remember, you must take *all* the nutrients which work together: vitamin D3, calcium, magnesium, and vitamin K2. The four work synergistically and are **best with fats** in the tummy. **K and D are fat soluble,** while calcium and magnesium will digest better with food in the stomach. Complete information on the supplements in *Mybyble* article "HEART PALPITATIONS".

CLOSE YOUR EYES IN ORDER TO FOCUS
Wiggle the Toothbrush, Visualization

Close your eyes when doing boring, repetitive tasks, such as brushing your teeth. With the eyes open, one tends to hurry through a task. With the eyes closed, one relaxes and can more properly attend to the task. For example, **never look in the mirror** while **brushing** your **teeth**. It causes you to rush. Turn your back to the mirror, close your eyes, and brush properly (which means angling the brush bristles into the gumline and *wiggling* the brush; **never** scrub the teeth or brush back and forth—this harms the enamel).

When you are on the slant board or you invert your body (see "Exercise"), also close your eyes. And when doing your neck exercise (See "Neck"), it will go more efficiently with your eyes closed (and turning on something that you enjoy: music, news?). When one exercises the arms, for example, if the eyes are closed and one *visualizes* the arm muscles toning and tightening, the brain can transport that thought to the muscles. I have read several times about visualizing. *The brain is very powerful.* It can accomplish much more than just thinking. It is a force that can support your actions.

When you do your deep breathing exercise, close your eyes and visualize that air coming in through your nose, going right down to the bottom of your stomach, and "blowing up a balloon" (see "Breathing").

Would you like to know what is behind this "close your eyes" concept? We all take in images through our eyes. There are three personality types: One takes in very few images; this person is mostly concerned with him/herself. Two sees what is going on and takes in those images. But Three is a **very** aware person who is bombarded all day by images even from his peripheral vision. For any person, closing the eyes for certain tasks will allow better concentration, focusing, and visualizing of the successful completion of the task or exercise.

DISTILLED WATER FOR CLEANING SPOTS

I was taking a prime minister to a breakfast in his honor at NASDAQ Stock Market headquarters in New York. He would also ring the opening buzzer and have press interviews.

Just before leaving the hotel, he brushed against something and got a big dirt spot on his suit jacket. I called engineering (machinery always uses distilled water [Why? For the same reason that it is good for spot cleaning and **not** leaving a ring: it has no inorganic minerals or contaminants which are **what** leave the ring! Thus, machinery needs pure water without minerals that clog up the works!]) and, bingo, got a gallon of distilled water sent up.

I set his jacket over a big bath towel and, using a clean washcloth and distilled water, dabbed and dabbed at the spot. It came out beautifully as distilled water leaves no ring because it contains no inorganic minerals.

I then used a blow dryer to dry the damp area.

The prime minister was amazed and said, "My dear Carole Lynn, if you ever write a book, this certainly should be in it!"

* * *

I have used distilled water on silk and just about every fabric. I have cleaned collars, cuffs, ties, marks on scarves, men's suits, and many other apparel items.

* * *

Sometimes a spot also needs a bit of Ivory soap, and I always use only the distilled water with the soap. Then I sop the soap out of the fabric with clear distilled water. On very special care, delicate garments, I have put the oxygen-based cleaner OxiClean into distilled water, stirred it, waited until it was dissolved, and then patted it into the stain (always placing the garment or item on top of a clean white terry cloth or towel); and then after the OxiClean solution does its work, I dab the spot with clear distilled water and, finally using another clean white terry cloth or Turkish towel, pat as much water out as possible. I then place the item on top of a large terry towel, smooth it into shape, and allow it to dry flat.

Always use a clean white cloth for the cleaning, and always set the item on top of a white Turkish or terry towel. You never want to risk a color dye from a towel transferring to your garment (as unlikely as that sounds, it happened to me once). Then **use a dry terry cloth** to help dry the fabric.

Certainly do not use more distilled water than necessary. With delicate fabrics, one wants to limit how much water or soap one uses. Use just enough to get the job done. One can also **test** the distilled water on an unseen section of the item just to be reassured that it will dry perfectly.

* * *

If you are spot cleaning a **washable** fabric, you **can** use soap and regular water for the spot. **Then,** in order to prevent a **ring** as the spot dries, use distilled water to finish off the cleaning process. Get rid of the tap-water-and-soap residue with distilled water, and use a clean terry cloth to dry up as much of the fabric as possible. Pat to absorb water. Do not rub.

* * *

To recap: How many of us have tried to clean a spot on a tie, blouse, trousers, or anything with tap water only to have that dreaded ring remain?

Distilled water is the answer. I have successfully spot-cleaned every garment including ones that say Dry Clean Only.

DISTILLED WATER INFORMATION

To clean any atomizer, use **distilled** water. Put the distilled water into the atomizer, and spray over and over until the spray is clear. Distilled water contains no inorganic matter. That is why most engineering departments have it on hand to use in machinery. It will not clog the mechanisms.

I use distilled water in my iron. See previous *Mybyble* article "Distilled Water for Cleaning Spots" on fabrics. It leaves no ring!

DIGESTION/INDIGESTION NUTRITION

Hydrochloric Acid, Digestive Enzymes

People know almost nothing about proper digestion. Nutrition should be taught starting in grade school, but while we grow up memorizing treaties from old wars, we are taught nothing about maintaining healthy bodies.

Children would benefit *so* greatly from proper nutrition which provides true nourishment from whole nutrients, good bowel movements, solid sleep, and adequate attention spans.

Adults, however, are the ones who wind up with stomach trouble, and they run for antacids. Most indigestion, though, is from a *lack* of **hydrochloric acid** in the stomach and also a *lack* of sufficient digestive enzymes. Suppressing the natural production of stomach acid is what causes most people's digestive woes. It is that acid which is necessary for digestion, and it is digestion which takes nutrients from foods eaten in order to nourish the body. When the stomach cannot digest food, the body winds up showing you that something is missing with **symptoms:** weak, splitting, or peeling fingernails; dry skin; hair or scalp problems; calluses on sides of heels; cracking heels; heartburn; and much more (all of which other *Mybyble* articles discuss). These are **not** normal signs of aging. These are **not** end results. These **are** symptoms alerting you to problems that need to be addressed and can be solved.

Dr. Bruce West writes thoroughly about the need for hydrochloric acid in *Health Alert* and how to test yourself to see if you have insufficient stomach acid. Read further in this article to see what I use for digestion.

Digestive Enzymes

We are born with a finite number of digestive enzymes. How well we take care of ourselves determines how long our supply lasts. Excessive drinking, non-nutritious foods, drugs, and poor eating habits (including improper food combining) will deplete the enzyme supply more quickly. Somewhere, though, between the ages of twenty-five and thirty (approximately), one should start supplementing the body's dwindling supply, and by fifty, the body certainly will need a digestive enzyme (and hydrochloric acid) boost!

Gas, belching, bloating, heartburn, diarrhea, and other body symptoms are all related to poor digestion.

Tip: Itching in the middle of one's back is a symptom of needing digestive enzymes and hydrochloric acid.

Guidance: *Acid reflux* is a symptom (almost always) of too <u>little</u> stomach acid, not too much. One should not suppress it but supplement it. Read further in article for "How Do I Know If I Have Too Little Stomach Acid?"

Tips for Better Digestion

Tip: If you have indigestion (and if you are at home), invert your body. Every once in a while even I do not have perfect digestion (especially when business stresses take over), and I swing onto my slant board and lie backward. The relief is almost immediate.

First of all, your organs are all going into their correct places. Secondly, you are taking pressure off the stomach and intestines and removing the effects of gravity.

When I am on a business trip and my stomach gets upset, I lie on the carpet of my hotel bedroom (on top of a nice, thick bath towel) and put my legs up on the bed. Then I raise up my pelvis in order to get a direct slant from knee to neck. It is very soothing. One can also lie on the bed and put one's feet on the wall above the headboard. Both of these positions can be used at home, too.

Tip: Patting (and even circular patting) the back between the shoulder blades helps relieve indigestion. It is where the nerve endings from the stomach all convene. It also helps the stomach to produce more hydrochloric acid. Dr. West once wrote a wonderful article about how this patting helped his grandmother cure her digestion problems.

Tip: Never eat potatoes and meat (see article "Food Combining") during the same meal. If you want potatoes, eat them as a main course and only with vegetables. Why? The stomach uses different digestive juices (enzymes) to digest protein and carbohydrates. It cannot digest both simultaneously. This results in food *not* being digested, nutrition lost, and an upset system.

Tip: Do not eat fruit as a dessert. Fruit should only be eaten on an empty stomach. The best time of day to eat fresh fruit and gain all its nutrient value is first thing in the morning. If fruit is eaten during the day, it should be at least two (preferably three) hours after an earlier meal. Why? Because ***fruit eaten on top of other food will rot that food*** in the stomach and prevent the digestion of nutrients in that food which would nourish the body, and also *it will delay elimination.* Instead of the digestive process taking twelve to twenty-four hours (and many times to seventy-two hours or longer, depending upon what was eaten; steak, for example, can take three to five days to digest and eliminate while food made with white flour takes a long time to digest and eliminate; fruits and vegetables [eaten separately and combined correctly] which are rich in fiber can be digested easily), that load of mismatched food will take thirty hours and longer to eliminate depending upon a person's system and how much food is sitting, now putrefying, and awaiting elimination. Healthy elimination of a properly combined meal should take twelve to twenty-four hours from eating a food to eliminating it as waste, but other food elimination can, indeed, take seventy-two hours. **Tip:** To see how long your digestive process and elimination take, drink some beet juice or eat four red beets. Beets tend to give a red hue to the stool, and you can judge how many hours your elimination took.

Personal Note: One of the early books in my life that had great impact was the first *Fit for Life* book by Harvey and Marilyn Diamond. It impressed upon me the need for proper **food combining** and the **disastrous results for the body when one combines incompatible foods**—incompatible in that they cannot be digested by the body at the same time.

This book provided an answer to my dilemma: I would have a meal at a restaurant and feel fine. Then, instead of a lovely chocolate cake, I would end the meal with a bowl of strawberries and unsweetened whipped cream. After that, my stomach felt just awful. It felt stuffed, and my abdomen was terribly uncomfortable (even if I did not have whipped cream; I tried eliminating that too). I was only thirty-three years old and knew that I was in good health. My dilemma was, Why was my stomach so sick when I had healthy strawberries? *Fit for Life* solved the problem. Fruit cannot be digested on top of other food, and it also halts the digestion of the food under it. After that, I enjoyed my cake and never had that difficulty again. See *Mybyble* article "Food Combining".

What Digestive Supplements Do I Take?

Everything that I mention here is in the "Source List" as well as additional comments. I have refined my digestives over many years due to my continuous reading on health issues and product evolvement. This protocol has helped many people, and I revamp it depending upon their individual needs. *Do not feel overwhelmed.* Start slowly, write things down, reread this article in a couple of days, take control of your health, and suddenly your supplement routine will be just that—routine!

Douglas Laboratories (www.douglaslabs.com)

1. Lipanase (pancreatic enzymes)
   Take one at the start of lunch, dinner, and also at any other big meals.

2. Vegetarian Enzyme
   Take one tablet (they are tiny tablets) at the start of **every** meal.

3. Betaine Plus
   I take one before breakfast, one before lunch (except if it is a big luncheon at a restaurant, then two), and two before dinner (along with items 1 and 2 above). This capsule contains betaine hydrochloride and pepsin which are critical to breaking down your food for digestion. People who get acid reflux, discomfort, gas, et al., are usually suffering from **a <u>deficiency</u> of digestive acids in the stomach**, and if they take mistakenly an acid *suppressant*, they compound the problem!

These three items will support properly digesting food *and other supplements* and getting the nutritional value from what is ingested! It is so important to remember that if digestion is impaired, supplements will not be digested. If the juices necessary for digestion are lacking, it is useless to take supplements.

P.S. You will notice **improvement in your nail growth** from these digestives; in particular, from betaine hydrochloride. Peeling, splitting, or soft nails can be a symptom of a <u>lack</u> of betaine hydrochloride (<u>*too little*</u> acid in the stomach as opposed to *too much*!).

Tip: **One huge symptom of the body needing digestive help is diarrhea!** Aside from gas, belching, heartburn, itching, sometimes back pain, et al., it is diarrhea which shows that the food taken in is being sent directly through the system *without being digested* and is eliminated as diarrhea.

There are two other digestives that I use for digestion:

A-F Betafood from Standard Process (see "Source List"). This product supports the normal processing of dietary fats, healthy bowel function, bile production in the liver and healthy bile flow in the gallbladder, and helps maintain healthy levels of fat in the liver. I take one tablet (with the others listed above) before lunch and one before dinner. If I am dining in a restaurant, I take two tablets before the meal. I have always found that A-F Betafood, combined with the other digestives, gives me better digestion.

Zypan, from Standard Process, combines pancreatin, pepsin, and betaine hydrochloride to facilitate healthy digestion. This tablet is one-third the strength of the Douglas Labs capsule Betaine Plus. Therefore, when I have a minimal snack, I just take one Zypan and one Vegetarian Enzyme tablet. It is not necessary to take the stronger capsule.

HOW DO I KNOW IF I HAVE TOO LITTLE STOMACH ACID?

If you are trying to determine what strengths of Zypan or Betaine Plus are best for your body, you could buy the small bottle of Zypan first. Try one tablet before a meal. If that goes well, then try two tablets. Finally, try three tablets. ***Your body will let you know*** if it has enough betaine hydrochloride by the stomach producing a slight burning sensation.

Tip: If you get any burning and you want to quickly get rid of it rather than wait for it to pass, place a quarter of a teaspoon of caraway seeds under your tongue or to the side of the mouth. Saliva will wet the seeds, and they will produce juices that will calm the stomach. Swallow the juice as it is produced from the saliva on the seeds. Once the seeds are nice and soft, chew them and swallow. See *Mybyble* article "Caraway Seeds." Over your lifetime, you will be thankful for this tip many times. **Caraway is the great stomach calmer as well**

as being healing for gums. (I also love rye bread with caraway seeds. Yes, those small black seeds are called caraway.)

Caraway will calm an upset stomach in an airplane or on a boat, and it is safe for those who are PREGNANT.

Note that I take two Betaine Plus before a major meal. That is equal in strength to six Zypan. It works perfectly for me. I have tested the amount and found that when I took more, I got a slight burning sensation. Hence, proof that I was taking the right dose for me.

EXERCISES/TONING
For Which You Do **Not** Need to Buy Equipment

There are a few exercises for toning the neck/face, back of arms, and eye area that can be done at home, in the office, or when traveling. They are the **best** exercises that I have ever found which **do not entail buying equipment**.

BACK OF ARMS (underarm flab)

The first exercise is for the underside of the upper arm just below the armpit. This area is almost impossible to tone specifically except with this exercise. It is so unpleasant to see yourself (look in a mirror) waving good-bye to someone and see that underarm shaking.

In the room where you want to do this exercise, find a sturdy chair (you do not want the chair to tip forward; the seat should be just above your knees) or radiator (one which has a flat-topped surrounding cover which is about as high as above your knees). On either one, place a folded terry towel in order to cushion your hands. Turn your back to the chair or radiator, reach down and place your hands on top and fingers over the edge, and do arm bends. Keep your hands directly behind your body, not off to the sides. Fingers should be curved down over the front of the object supporting you.

IMPORTANT: You will **bend the elbows**, not your shoulders or arms. Just have the elbows release in order to lower the upper arm; then lock the elbows to straighten your arms. In the straightened position, hold to the count of three. Then release the elbows to lower the upper arm. In other words, it is the inside of your **upper** arm that is controlling the effort and thus toning. Additionally, the lower arm gets a workout just from supporting the effort. It is actually supporting the weight of the upper body as one goes up and down. Therefore, it is a functional, weight-bearing exercise for the lower arm.

I am five feet eight inches, and I favor using a radiator that comes just to the top of my knee. When I travel, I look for something in the room of similar height.

SUGGESTION: If you want to see exactly what muscles are being used in exercises (and a mirror is not available), ask a friend to do the exercise so you can observe. Also (for example, with arm or leg exercises), you can *feel* different muscle exertion if you slightly alter the position of the arms or legs. You are able to *feel* other muscles take over. Then you will realize why a specific position is dictated for certain toning or other benefits.

EYES

The muscles of the upper eyelid and just below the eye need strengthening as we age (and even earlier for some). I noticed that the skin around my eyes was not as taut as it once was. Also, when I blew my nose too hard, the muscle under my left eye twitched terribly.

Two exercises completely helped. ***Look in the mirror*** until you master these. Then you can do them anywhere: while on your slant board (or on the floor with legs up on the bed), every time you go to the bathroom (take a couple of extra minutes and do some isometrics while looking in the mirror), on the train while commuting, or anywhere that you can take a few moments for your health. **With isometrics, the effect is cumulative. One does not have to do an extensive set all at one time. They can be done several times a day, and the results are cumulative.**

1. UNDER EYES: Put your lips in a position of saying "ew" (like "pee-yew," not as round as "oh," but "ew"). You are then

going to move the muscles beneath the eyes <u>in</u> toward the nose. Pretend that you are trying to squeeze the bridge of your nose with the muscles beneath your eyes. Every bit helps, but two or three sets of ten is most useful (squeeze, hold, release). While doing this, keep your eyes open; do not squint or frown. Look straight into the mirror until you master these isometrics.

2. ABOVE EYELIDS: Close your eyes. Now, <u>keeping them closed,</u> try to open them. (Do <u>not</u> open them.) Using muscles above the eyelid, pull up. And do <u>not</u> raise your eyebrows.

Only a few will help, but two or three sets of ten is most effective.

I found this isometric to particularly strengthen my whole eye, including the eyeball.

NECK AND FACE

While lying flat on your back, lift head no more than a quarter of an inch. Lift **only** to that degree where gravity is pulling you down and you are trying to pull up. You will feel your head vibrate at that instant where gravity is pulling you back. Again, the head will only be an eighth to a quarter of an inch off the ground or slant board. Hold to a count of three to five seconds. Put head back down. Repeat.

Do this for as long as you have time in order to strengthen neck muscles—in particular, the front of the neck—as well as tone the face. You can also turn your head to both sides and lift-and-lower in order to specifically exercise those muscles.

This exercise can also be done while lying inverted. I like to have some good music playing. I know just how many songs will take me through the routine.

The EYES and the NECK/FACE isometrics can also be done while lying on the slant board (or other partial inversion). Not only do you have blood flow nourishing the brain and face, but you are accomplishing other productive tasks <u>with your eyes closed.</u> See tips in articles "Close Your Eyes" and "Hang Upside Down."

FUNNY BONE (ELBOW) and ISOMETRICS
Nerve Damage, Weak Muscles, Tendons and Ligaments, Improved Bustline and Thighs
Used in Scoliosis Treatment

Years ago I badly banged my elbow—the funny bone. There was nothing humorous about it. Months went by; doctors and physical therapists (in those days I still visited doctors albeit rarely) were visited to no avail. The elbow was so bad that at certain times I cradled it with my other hand while holding the bad arm folded over my chest.

Heading to a business meeting at 7:00 am, and in agony, I suddenly remembered that years before, I heard that isometrics help nerve damage as well as strengthen the muscles, tendons, and ligaments. Since I was not driving the car, I immediately grasped my fingers together (one hand pulling the other) and pulled, holding to the count of twenty. Release. Repeat. Unbelievably, I felt relief. After several sets of pulls, I then did pushes, placing palms together, fingers pointed upward, elbows out, chest held high. The position of the hands, arms, and elbows is specific: arms chest-high, elbows out, chest out / shoulders back.

Every time I had pain during the day, I ran to a ladies room and exercised. If no one was around, I used the edge of an open door, grasping my fingers around to pull and alternately pressing palms against either side of the door to push. The relief was immediate and sustained.

As days went by, the isometrics caused the pain to diminish and finally disappear.

I suggest that you **start the isometrics undressed and looking in a mirror**. I use my bathroom mirror. Once you master them, you can do them fully dressed anywhere: **sitting** in the car, on a commuter train or bus, while watching television, or even taking a break at the computer. You can squeeze and release your **thighs** at the same time you do your arms and eyes (see previous article), or, when sitting, put your feet together, knees splayed outward, tighten **the thighs**, and press as though you are going to close your knees but do ***not***; again, it is the tension that strengthens and tones.

I enjoy going out on my terrace in the morning as the 9:00 am sun shines down (or even on a cloudy day). I breathe in several times and do my arm and eye isometrics while getting vitamin D from the sun. This is a multibeneficial activity.

The **reason to start doing them undressed** (inside one's home by a mirror) is because **you will see (in the mirror) exactly what muscles are being worked**. You should also **turn sideways** and look in the mirror to see how the pushes and pulls cause muscles in your chest, side, and back to tighten and raise up. They go back to positions that they had when the body was young (before gravity exerted its force). This can be recaptured. Isometric exercise is using tension in order to build strength and tone. **These isometrics will also improve the bustline** by firming and building. Females of any age will especially benefit. *Personal Note:* I first learned this when I was fourteen years old, and I did this isometric like crazy in my quest to build my bust (à la my teenage friends).

Isometrics not only treat an injury but also build and tone the body part being addressed. See article "Scoliosis." There are two other isometrics for the arms, chest, and back in addition to the two above (pulling, pushing). If one does a sequence of all four exercises, the varied muscles—front, back, inside/outside of arms, chest, sides—will be worked. **The other two are as follows:**

- First isometric: Elbows out, arms even with chest, chest up, shoulders back, and fingertips (not palms) touching and pointing up. Then press to the count of twenty. Release. Do five sets, ten, or twenty. Alternatively, you can do five sets several times daily.

- The second isometric of these is same position as above. Fingertips touching. But you reverse the hands and have the fingertips pointing downward. Press to the count of twenty. Release. Repeat.

When you view yourself in a mirror, it is very instructive to see which muscles move: in arms, chest, side, and back. It shows what is being worked. Once this is mastered, the isometrics can be done anywhere you wish (as I wrote before). If you close your eyes, you can visualize what you saw in the mirror. This enhances the exercise. Again, watch in the mirror, and be aware of which muscles move to each of these four isometrics. Note not only the side, back, and front but **also which muscles in the entirety of the arms and torso** are being worked.

Remember that while you do these isometrics, you can also do the eye isometrics which I describe in the article "Exercises/Toning: Eyes". While doing isometrics myself, I also tighten and release my thighs as well as hold in the stomach muscles and raise the rib cage as I do my pushes and pulls.

In reading about isometrics, one learns that the bonus is that its **effects are cumulative!** Unlike normal exercising where you only benefit with a certain number of repetitions, isometric benefits accumulate. If one does some pushes and pulls now and a few later and more tomorrow, the benefit is cumulative. Incredible. Try one or two; over a few weeks, you can develop a routine that focuses on areas that are important to you.

Personal Note: This article started with mention of the funny bone. Please, in the future, every time you bang your funny bone (and you will) and then get immediate relief with the isometrics taught here, please smile and think of *Mybyble*.

REBOUNDING ON MINITRAMPOLINE

Every single cell of the body is toned as you leave gravity on your bounce up—no matter how tiny the bounce. This alone is sufficient reason to rebound. It frees up your whole body. Systems within the body, I feel, rebalance themselves. Jumping clears sinuses, relieves gas (causes the body to expel gas), and benefits lymph glands as well as skin, other organs, eyes, and muscles.

I first used a trampoline in gym class in high school. That was a big trampoline, and members of the class took turns spotting for one another, because whoever was jumping had to have spotters on all sides of the trampoline in case she misstepped and toppled sideways or backward. The spotters all had their arms up in order to catch and push back the jumper. I even learned to do a summersault in the air on the trampoline. Fantastic!

At my home now, I have a minitrampoline (also called a rebounder). It is only three feet in diameter, can fold up, or—as I keep it—lying against a wall when not in use. But there is one *critical* rule: when you jump, you must keep your eyes focused on a single point approximately eight to ten feet away, and it should be level with your eyes. You should not be looking up or down, just straight ahead. That point keeps you balanced. It keeps you from toppling over. Many minitrampolines come with instructions, but this rule is the most important one!

Start slowly until you get the hang of it. You can even sit down and bounce. Some rebounders have handles (removable handrails). These can be used until one feels competent to jump freely. And **remember to breathe!** It is a funny thing, but when one is rebounding, there is a tendency not to breathe or to breathe shallowly. Just breathe naturally.

I jump first thing in the morning. First, I do sixty scissors: sending my arms up in the air over my head while legs are going out and in. Then I do a walking step (forward and back) while pumping my arms. After forty of those, I send my legs on a diagonal (call it 8:00 and 2:00 out to the sides followed by 10:00 and 4:00), twenty of each, arms still pumping, using a nice swinging motion as I would if I was power walking outdoors. Finally, I send my legs straight out to either side (9:00 and 3:00) with arms pumping. I do twenty of each of these. Then I gently bounce for about thirty seconds which calms the body, and **this is very important**. You never leap off the rebounder because balance may not be steady. Just bounce in place before *carefully* stepping off the rebounder. I exit the trampoline and attend to something for about three to five minutes and then do the routine again. I do this three times.

Before bed I always jump but only for a short routine. **Years ago I read, "If you walk up and down a flight of stairs before going to bed, at the end of one year—as long as you do not increase your food intake—you will lose seven pounds".** I do not want to lose any pounds, but maintenance is a good thing. Since I do not have a staircase, I consider doing a certain amount of jumping equal to a flight of stairs. In this case, it is three minutes or a drop longer.

There is a very good book by Dr. Morton Walker, DPM, called *Jumping for Health: A Guide to Rebounding Aerobics*, which was written in 1989. It is most informative.

The minitrampolines need to be replaced every few years depending upon how often they are used as well as a person's weight. Over the years, I have bought them mostly from Walmart. They have ranged in price from $29.99 to $39.99. It pays to check the discount stores when one is buying. Often there are sales. See "Source List" at end.

CROSS CRAWL
Memory, Coordination, Brain Function, Mental Agility, Balance

Serves as an Afternoon Refresher/ Pick-Me-Up in the Office or at Home

The brain is a powerful instrument. It is not only for thinking. Do you know that it is the brain that actually *sees*? Eyes receive the visual information while the brain processes this information into useful images.

Memory and coordination change or deteriorate with age or illness. With age, it is not *due to age* that the brain is not functioning as it did earlier but to the care that has been accorded the body, or, shall we say, to the care *lacking* in the body. The extended lifespan, as is mentioned elsewhere in *Mybyble*, delivers burdens unknown in the past. We need to use nutrition—meaning whole food and supplements—as well as exercise to support the body and all its parts which were not originally designed to survive for ninety or one hundred years.

The cross crawl is another great and unique gift from *Mybyble*. **Cross crawl exercises are a way to reprogram the brain, the nervous system, the spinal muscles, and various body systems so that they work optimally together**. Cross crawl can be used preventively or therapeutically. To **keep the brain, memory, and coordination toned and maintained**, one can use cross crawl. For someone in the throes of any kind **of mental issue—and that includes Alzheimer's** disease—the cross crawl can be of great benefit.

Does someone you know **get up during the night** to urinate and become **disoriented** trying to make their way to the bathroom? It is a **symptom** that the brain needs toning. I put someone on cross crawl, and he no longer crashes into furniture or closet doors trying to get to the bathroom during the night.

What Is Cross Crawl?

When we walk, the natural position and rhythm is right arm and right leg forward followed by the left arm and leg. With the cross crawl, you swing the right arm forward with the *left* leg. You use the leg on the opposite side from the arm.

You are thinking right now, "Oh, sure. Easy." Go and try it. It is a total contradiction to our normal walking pattern. To get started, put your foot forward, then put the opposite arm forward. Now, slowly walk, and keep alternating. If you do this slowly, you will pick up the pattern. This can also be done walking in place (standing in one spot).

Cross crawl can also be accomplished walking backward. See the following article "Walking Backward" for complete information on this fascinating topic.

The world's aging population continues to grow. About fourteen years ago, I presented a program on Bloomberg Radio: "The

Extended Lifespan, and Are You Prepared for It *Financially*?" (See *Mybyble* article.) Take the subject fourteen years later and ask, "The extended lifespan, and are you prepared for it *healthwise*?" In particular, are you keeping your brain engaged?

With cross crawl patterning, we **rebuild and reset nerve function and regain stability**. This is extremely beneficial following trauma of any kind. Cross crawl walking is one of the easiest ways to **activate the brain and nervous system** in order to give it the proper motor and sensory stimuli it needs to take care of bodily functions in order to either prevent or rehabilitate problems.

An important point is that one never does this exercise to exhaustion. It is only done until *early* fatigue. Additionally, the maximum benefits from cross crawl are from executing the motions slowly. The brain benefits most from *wide range* of motion which provides more stimuli to the brain. Therefore, focus on the movements and not on speed.

Cross crawl can also be done sitting in a chair. Thrust one foot forward while swinging the opposite arm upward. This is very good for in the office or anytime that a pick-me-up is needed. *It reinvigorates the brain.* This is also a *good way for someone who is ill* to start accumulating the benefits of cross crawl. One can also move the limbs sideways as well as out to an angle (on a diagonal), all from a seated position.

Cross crawl can also be done down on all fours in a crawling position. One can also try cross crawling (whether upright or on all fours) with the eyes closed in order to improve balance; however, you should have someone standing beside you, as maintaining balance with the eyes closed is difficult.

Amongst other articles and sites, www.headbacktohealth.com has detailed information. Go to its Index, and click on Cross Crawl.

If you have a minitrampoline, please refer to the previous article and the directions in which I exercise my arms and legs on the rebounder for walking and the diagonal. One can (on the rebounder) also do the cross crawl. Again, start slowly. Focus your eyes forward on a single point. When I first started the cross crawl on the rebounder, it took a few minutes to master this reverse pattern. Now, I do my normal routine followed by a complete cross crawl routine. I also do both before bedtime but briefly.

Many people will find that it takes more than a few minutes to master cross crawl (the longer it takes to master it, <u>the more your brain needs it</u>!); however, the benefits to your health are significant. **THIS IS A TIP OF A LIFETIME!**

WALKING BACKWARD
Tone the Abdomen

WALKING FORWARD

Walking forward normally and briskly is great exercise. Swing those arms <u>**above**</u> the head, and (as taught to me by a doctor in Singapore) after four to eight minutes, depending upon whether one is walking on any incline, you can be burning calories up to four times faster than when not swinging those arms over the head. It also depends upon whether one is carrying light weights or not. I have used the light weights; however, I prefer the freedom of swinging my arms with my hands free. Always remember to never clench the fist (that is stressful to the body). The ***over-the-head swing also firms the tummy.***

Then I was introduced to **WALKING BACKWARD** from a health article about thirty years ago. This is especially beneficial for ***toning the abdomen***. What a joy, and how liberating to do this on a beach. Wherever the location, I walk backward keeping my eyes focused on a distant point in order to maintain a straight walking path and, again, swinging my arms straight up and above my head.

I also have a treadmill in my home which provides an incline. This is so useful for both forward and backward walking.

STAIR CLIMBING

Stairs offer another exercise alternative. If one lives in an apartment building or in a private home with a staircase, there is a built-in advantage. The two ways here to exercise are going up stairs and going down. You laugh, but there is a point to be made.

TONING: If you want to tone the legs and lower body, you want to walk *down* steps! Yes, down. Here is the lesson: What is the hardest step for a little child to learn because it needs such muscle control? The answer: Walking *down* steps without holding on to anything.

If one is seeking to tone, you will go down steps in order to maximize using those muscles and thus toning them. *AND* **the slower you go**, the more you are toning because it takes muscle control to slow the pace.

WEIGHT LOSS AND CARDIOVASCULAR WORKOUT: Going *up* stairs provides a cardio workout. If you *pump your arms*, you burn still more fat and tone the upper body. Also, a *quicker pace* causes more fat to burn.

HEART PALPITATIONS, ARRHYTHMIAS
Cough to Get Your Heart Beating
(With Notes on Osteoporosis and Heart Disease)
RESTLESS LEG SYNDROME

Most people, at some time or other, have an irregular heartbeat or palpitations; some would describe this as "my heart fluttering". **_Cough_** to get the heart beating again in proper rhythm.

Naturally, this does not mean to cough one's brains out. It means to cough quickly from the chest. This should restart a proper rhythm.

Three personal notes: *First Note:* I was on an airplane, and we had just taken off. The gentleman to my right suddenly sat up, dropped his magazine, and put his right hand on the window. He was struggling to breathe. I quickly placed my right hand on his left arm to calm him and asked, "Is it your heart? Is it fluttering?" I just had the feeling that that was the problem. He quickly nodded yes, and I told him, "Cough!" He looked at me frantically but also warily, and I said, "Trust me. Cough from your chest. It will reset your heart rhythm." He did. He could not believe it and said to me, "Thank you. Thank you. I am in your debt. **You should write a book!**" I do hope that that gentleman reads this article.

Secondly, I did a television interview regarding finance on ***The Woman's Connection*** **® (www.womans-connection.com)**. Near the end of the show, the host (Ms. Barrie-Louise Switzen) said that she knew that aside from my being financially savvy, I was very knowledgeable regarding health. She asked me if I could offer the audience one health tip. I offered this one ("Cough to Get Your Heart Beating"). Barrie-Louise later told me that the responding audience cared more about the *health* tips than the financial ones!

Thirdly, I have seen coughing stabilize the heartbeat while someone awaited an ambulance. He managed to do quick coughs, and the paramedic said, "Lucky you knew this, sir. It could save a lot of folks."

Now, back to the article. Of course, if this heart fluttering (skipping beats) is a very frequent occurrence, it would possibly indicate a nutrient deficiency. There are two sets of nutrients that, if deficient, can cause this: first, calcium, magnesium, vitamin D3, and vitamin K2 (these four work synergistically); and, secondly, the B vitamins. Note that either of these two vitamin groups can also be what is deficient if one has **RESTLESS LEG SYNDROME.** Supplement with one group first in order to see the results; then the other, if necessary. Finally, try both groups.

First, let me describe the need for magnesium, calcium, D3, and K2 which work together. Do not take one without the other as that would create an imbalance. I buy Douglas Laboratories' Amino-Mag (200 mg) and Osteo-guard (microcrystalline calcium hydroxyapatite [MCHC]) (250 mg.), taking three Osteogard and four Amino-Mag, spread out from morning until dinner (for example, magnesium at 10:00 am, calcium at 12:00 noon, magnesium around 2:00 pm, calcium around 4:00 pm, calcium again just before dinner, and two magnesium, which relaxes the body, closer to bedtime). **IMPORTANT**: MCHC is an extremely bioavailable form of calcium, and it is well tolerated. Careful processing allows MCHC to retain all the bone minerals and organic residues intact and in their natural physiological ratios. This contributes to enhanced absorption and bone uptake. For those concerned with **osteoporosis,** British research showed that MCHC was uniquely found to not only prevent further bone loss but to restore mineral content.

Hydroxyapatite, a crystalline substance within the body, comprises nearly 50 percent of the body's bone mineral. Depending upon one's age and health needs, one might need more calcium and magnesium (perhaps one more of each item per day depending upon one's diet). Various articles indicate different dosages; however, Dr. Mercola (in his article "Magnesium-The Missing Link to Better Health") quotes a medical expert on magnesium who **indicates a 1:1 ratio between calcium and magnesium**. Hence, the four Amino-Mag and three Osteogard which provide close to a 1:1 ratio (800 mg to 750 mg.).

I use Douglas Laboratories' D3 (1,000 IU) and take one tablet five times daily with the Osteo-guard, calcium, and magnesium. One **always wants some fatty food in the stomach** (milk or cream from tea, butter, or another fatty food) when taking **vitamin D because it is fat soluble.** Numerous medical experts recommend 5,000 IUs daily as a maintenance dosage for those who are not getting D3 from the sun. I spread out the doses using five 1,000 IU tablets in order to maximize absorption.

Just an aside here: I write elsewhere in *Mybyble* that I take off two days per week from taking supplements as well as taking off the first week of every month. I feel that that allows my body some 'free' time (as well as "time off for good behavior").

As with vitamin D, it is the same situation with **vitamin K2. It is fat soluble.** I buy Ultra Vitamin K with Advanced K2 Complex (item no. NSI 7013470) from Vitacost because, in my opinion, it has a good mix of the different K segments. It took me a long time to find this particular vitamin K. As more and more research comes out, it is apparent that vitamin K2 is critical in its working with magnesium, calcium, and D3, and especially with calcium. Vitamin K2 helps move calcium into the proper areas of your body; for example, bones and teeth. If one takes supplemental D3, this increases the need for K2.

An excellent article describing this is by Dr. Mercola on Mercola.com: "Beyond Calcium and Vitamin D—How to Really Build Strong Bones". Currently, I take two K2 soft gels per day (at separate times in order to allow the body to fully digest and utilize it), and I take one K with my first calcium of the day and the second with my calcium just before dinner (and with fats in the tummy).

Secondly, there is the need for B vitamins and good fats (see article "Danger of Low-Fat/No-Fat Diets"), especially since people's diets have become so poor and devoid of necessary nutrients in that diets are loaded with sugar, incorrect fats (notice that I write "incorrect fats"; that is because good fats are extremely necessary for a healthy body; butter [preferably organic and cultured], raw organic nuts and seeds, organic meat/game/fowl/fish, organic coconut oil [on breads and toast or on pasta], high-lignan flax oil, nonprocessed cheese, and goat milk [such as Oak Knoll Goat Milk] are fats that contribute to and support a healthy body; see the "Source List"), and other unhealthy ingredients as well as **prescription drugs (most of which sap the body of many nutrients;** just read the information sheets that come with medications; they are a fright!). **Poor diets do not provide adequate B vitamins, and this stresses the heart**. Dr. Bruce West (who writes *Health Alert*) calls this "beriberi of the heart", and he has full articles on this as well as his protocol using Standard Process whole food-based products that enrich the heart and body and provide the missing nutrients naturally. Please see *Mybyble* article "Learn" for information on Dr. West.

I include a quote here because heart trouble is so prevalent, and there is no question but that this will help many people, if not save lives. A person would need to search far and wide to find this information. In the August 2013 *Health Alert* (volume 30, issue 8, pages 5 and 6), Dr. West writes:

> ". . . beriberi of the heart—a B-vitamin disease that paralyzes and cripples nerves and muscles—most

often in and around the heart. The lesson: millions of Americans suffer from what I call sub-clinical beriberi of the heart which mimics all kinds of heart disease, including congestive heart failure."

And he continues

"Most cardiac arrhythmias (abnormal heartbeats) are not a disease—no matter what name is given. Rather they are a symptom of a heart that is weakened by nutritional deficiencies and trying desperately to keep functioning by beating slower, faster, erratically, and in whatever fashion it can. Therefore, treating arrhythmias with drugs and even ablation (burning nerve sites in the heart) is generally futile."

He goes on to describe the Standard Process supplement protocol which he recommends.

Included in the Standard Process B vitamin group which I use are: Cataplex B, Cardio-Plus, and Vasculin (in particular, for my venous insufficiency). My doses of these products are for maintenance, while those needing a therapeutic regimen would follow stronger dosing and possibly additional nutrients. See "Source List" where I also mention Puritan's Pride Complete B (all in one caplet).

Hence, we are back to what I have written in *Mybyble* more than once: one must be careful not to treat the *symptom* but to *go to the cause* of the symptom. Symptoms are your body knocking on the 'door' in your head in order to beg for help. They are letting you know that there is some problem needing attention. Many times, it is a deficiency of a nutrient or the need for stronger-than-usual nutrient supplements.

URINE TO THE RESCUE
Cuts, Paper Cuts, Insect Bites, Rashes, Hives, Rosacea

Contains One's Own Human Growth Hormone!

There are several wonderful books on urine therapy. Until you try it—especially in an emergency—do not turn up your nose:

1. *Your Own Perfect Medicine* by Martha M. Christy, 1994
2. *The Golden Fountain: The Complete Guide to Urine Therapy* by Coen van der Kroon, 2001

These books introduce the world of urine therapy including drinking one's own urine (first urine of the morning, midstream) because, as research indicates, it benefits the immune system and has **antiviral, antibacterial, and antifungal activities as well as containing one's own human growth hormone!** *This* is the benefit that really caught my eye. Considering that people (as certain actors and actresses are written about doing this) travel to other countries in order to get injections of human growth hormone and take various medicaments that supposedly increase their human growth hormone, it was fascinating and edifying to read that one's own urine contains this.

Whether drinking the urine or using it on a rash or hive, one should use a clean cup (plastic or otherwise), and collect the midstream urine from the first urine of the day (for some folks, that will be in the middle of the night). I suggest having two or three cups on hand. Discard anything left (into the toilet) at night. Use two or three other fresh cups for the next morning. The used cups can be washed and reused. After all, **urine—from a healthy person—is a sterile and clean substance and bacteria-free**.

Tip for getting started: Put your finger into the urine in the cup, and then let **five drops** fall from your finger into your mouth just under the tongue. Those drops are immediately absorbed, and one avoids a gag reflex. You taste nothing, and those drops will actually benefit the body. Do this for many days, and increase the number of drops as you progress.

A good diet devoid of bad foods and drugs produces a light-color urine with no odor. Urine is a good indicator of whether one's diet is healthy.

Additionally, similar to our saliva, one's **urine contains healing enzymes**. You know when people get a cut on the finger and you see them lick it? That is because saliva contains healing enzymes. Many people do not **know** this; however, they instinctively lick the cut. Animals do, as well. Well, urine, too, contains these healing enzymes.

Paper cuts are particularly galling, as they are so tiny yet so hugely irritating. Put some urine on toilet tissue. Hold it onto the cut for a few moments. It heals the cut! Or, stick your finger into your urine stream, and let it work full strength. Just dab the wet finger dry with toilet tissue; the urine will already be working.

Insect bites, a sudden rash, and hives usually respond the same way. A friend of mine was stung in the foot by a stingray in the ocean when we were snorkeling and diving in Australia in Cairns. For lack of any other medicaments, in agony, and with his buddy yelling, "Pee on it!", he did. It worked. We never forgot this.

The premise is this: Our bodies hold the enzymes that can heal ourselves. They are in our urine. The healthier the person, the healthier is the urine. How do you think people who are stranded after an airplane crash survive? They must drink their <u>own</u> urine.

During a day at the office, just before an important meeting, on an airplane, or any time you get that inopportune cut, hive, or insect bite, try it. **It is easy, nontoxic, free, and worthwhile. It is, after all, your own urine.**

If you ever get something annoying by your eyelashes or any itching of the eyelid, use urine to clean the lids and upper and lower lashes. **(Stop saying "Yuck". Someday you will be glad that you know this).** Dab urine onto the edge of a tissue or a Q-tip and gently touch that to the affected spot. Keep the urine outside the eye; just along the outer area where there is itching or irritation.

This treatment works nicely when also using emu oil. After lightly putting the urine near the eye, once it dries one can, using a cotton swab, dab on a speck of emu oil to soothe the inflamed or itchy spot.

Personal Note: The apartment building in which I resided was having outdoor brick work done. The men would drill into the bricks, doing what is called point work. There was a terrace outside my bedroom and also the air-conditioner. The men failed to let me know to shut off the air-conditioner, and some bad air and debris came into the bedroom. The next day, I suddenly had a rash on my face, and it continued to get worse.

I was told that it was probably **rosacea**. The only thing that I could connect this to was that infected air coming into my bedroom. It was too coincidental. When I researched **rosacea, one particular article stood out because it said that this was a bacterial disease**. Well, I know that 3 percent hydrogen peroxide can be used to treat a bacterial infection, and I used it. It was indeed helpful but not a cure.

Quite a long time went by until I found four things that cured this rash which included pimple-like eruptions (which never healed from the middle but from the outer edges drying up):

1. My own urine. See the previous article regarding collecting midstream morning urine in a clean plastic cup. I used a Q-tip to dab the urine on the rash all day long. The urine worked in a totally different way than the peroxide. The urine <u>*drew out*</u> bacteria from inside. The tiny bump marks on my face reacted to the urine and sent out whatever was causing the condition. Each protrusion would look like a tiny white balloon. I learned quickly ***not*** to rub or pop these white balloons because that disrupted the healing process. When the urine had caused all the poison to be expelled from beneath the skin, the little white balloons simply became a flat crust and fell off. The skin underneath was fine.
2. Retin-A. A female doctor friend told me that Retin-A corrects skin problems. So, I got a prescription for all three strengths. I tested the weakest one first and then continued to the other two. The strongest was perfect. I put a ***<u>speck</u>*** on my finger and

would put this *infinitesimal* dot on top of any white balloons or bumps under my skin. The Retin-A got rid of them! The bumps receded while those white balloons dried up much more quickly. Remember, though, that I used less than a pinprick on top of each eruption. Retin-A is powerful. For me, it was a blessed healer.
3. Washing my face with organic virgin coconut oil from Omega Nutrition. See article in *Mybyble*. I stopped using soap and went to **this** coconut oil which not only nourishes the skin but is also antimicrobial. Therefore, whatever bacteria caused this condition, it was being zapped with the help of this coconut oil while leaving my skin silky smooth.
4. Using NutriBiotic Grapefruit Seed Extract, placing fifteen drops (therapeutic dose) three times daily in pure water, stirring, and drinking. I take my vitamins with this water. Many times I split up the dose, doing eight drops or six drops. In the end, though, it added up to forty-five drops per day. This was the final healing ingredient in my self-treatment. See the "Source List" for information.

Second Personal Note: While writing *Mybyble*, I went to change a lightbulb, and a jagged piece of metal jabbed into my right hand in the padding below the thumb. Lots of blood spurted, but my urine sealed it within two minutes. I always keep a plastic cup of morning urine in the bathroom. I dabbed urine (with a cotton swab) on this deep cut for four days at which time it was totally healed.

DEEP BREATHING
Cleanse System, Expel Polluted Air, Tone Cells, **Hot Flashes**

Years ago, I read in a health article that if there was one thing that the writer would do to maintain his health and enhance his whole body inside and out, it would be deep breathing. In recent years, I am again reading about the benefits of cleansing one's lungs of pollutants as well as energizing our cells. Sign up for "The Optimal Breathing Times" complimentary e-mail from Michael White at www.breathing.com.

Sitting, lying, standing, or on the slant board, you can deep breathe.

Always breathe in through the nose and out through the mouth. **Here is the key that most descriptions of breathing never tell you: Imagine that you are blowing up a balloon in your stomach.** Bring air in through the nose and direct it to your stomach (as low in the body as you can go). Your stomach should swell out as air enters; do *not* hold your stomach in. Take the air in slowly and steadily and let it rise (from filling the stomach) to move up into the lungs and feel them swell with air. When your body is truly oxygenated and full of air, your shoulders will rise!

Then exhale through the mouth, releasing the air from the upper lungs first and all the way down to the stomach which will then tighten and contract. **Doing this only ten times is beneficial.** It is easier to master this while lying down or partially inverted.

A second breathing cleanser is to take in air as described, then lower your chin to your chest, and <u>forcefully</u> exhale via mouth until your lungs are empty. Repeat.

This is especially good if you have been in a smoky room or other polluted or germy atmosphere. Expel that residue from the lungs. Replace it with clean air.

<u>**HOT FLASHES**</u>: This is mentioned separately in *Mybyble*; however, I repeat that deep breathing is one of the most balancing things that one can easily do in order to stabilize hot flashes. You do not even need the entire routine described above. Just **close** your eyes. Breathe in. **Hold** that breath. Release air through the mouth. It is those moments—while you **<u>hold that breath</u>**—that are so important. Empty your mind, hold your breath, eyes closed, and feel your body balancing and stabilizing.

FROZEN BREAD OR CAKE

If your bread is slightly dry or has been in the freezer, lightly spray water (preferably pure bottled water without fluoride or chlorine and other inorganic material) from an atomizer onto the bread or cake.

Zap in the microwave, and it is nice and freshened. You can even toast the bread for perfect toast. Try just ten seconds in the microwave. See if that is sufficient. I freeze my favorite bread which is **Alvarado Street Bakery (www.alvaradostreetbakery.com)** sprouted organic breads from California. They are available in many U.S. supermarkets. **It is being "sprouted" that gives the eater benefit of more protein, vitamins, and minerals** than from refined flour. I buy Alvarado's Multi-Grain, Barley, Rye, and Flax Seed as well as others. When frozen, I spray my bottled water on the edges of the bread as well as the center and then microwave for fourteen seconds. Then I toast it and use both Omega Nutrition Organic Virgin Coconut Oil and Organic Valley Cultured Unsalted Butter. I accompany my Alvarado toast with either raw, organic walnuts, pecans, cashews, and unpasteurized almonds, or, with raw, organic sunflower and pumpkin seeds. Note that I have always found my Alvarado bread to stimulate peristalsis.

If you do not have water in a mister or atomizer to spray on, simply dampen some paper towels or a cloth. Wrap the bread in it for a few moments. Then continue.

Pure bottled water in an atomizer (mister) will not clog up the atomizer the way tap water gradually will (because of minerals in the tap water).

DISTILLED WATER

To clean any atomizer, use **distilled** water. Put the distilled water into the atomizer, and spray over and over until the spray is clear. Distilled water contains no inorganic matter. That is why most engineering departments have it on hand to use in machinery. It will not clog the mechanisms. I use distilled water in my iron. *Mybyble* has another article "Distilled Water for Cleaning Spots" on fabrics.

SELF-TANNING LOTIONS
Surgical Rubber Gloves to the Rescue

Use rubber gloves to apply self-tanning lotion. You will protect your palms and nails from discoloring and be able to more evenly rub it on.

One can use any type of rubber glove; however, I prefer a thin one. Go to Home Depot, Lowe's, or a surgical supply store, and buy the thin surgical gloves (in a large-quantity box; they even come in colors, aside from clear).

PROTECT NAILS AND HANDS
PACKING, CLEANING, CHORES, GROCERY SHOPPING
Use Surgical (Rubber) Gloves

Paper cuts and destroyed manicures are so annoying . . . as are germs. Wear surgical gloves when you are packing, cleaning, doing any household or office chores, or even when grocery shopping.

I buy turquoise-colored gloves. Of course, there are clear ones, white ones, and nude. I happily wear the turquoise one when shopping. Everyone asks me, "How did you ever think of such a clever idea?" Even men have complimented this use of gloves, and one gentleman said, "Hey! I must tell my wife about that. She's always nicking her nails when shopping. You should write a tips book!"

REMOVING NAIL POLISH

Thin rubber gloves are perfect when removing nail polish. Why get polish remover all over your skin from a saturated cotton ball? The glove is so protective.

FUR

Fur hats and collars of fur coats pick up oils from the skin. Sprinkle talcum powder on the edges that come into contact with the skin (after each wearing), and use a soft-bristle brush to brush out the powder. The talc will remove accumulated oils.

CAROLE LYNN STEINER

LIPSTICK ON TEETH

A lovely woman. An attractive smile. Oh no! Lipstick on her teeth!

Simple to prevent this: Upon completing the application of lipstick, purse your lips together in an O position; stick your finger in and out (wipe on a tissue), in and out again (wipe). Your finger removes all the lipstick from the inner part of the lips that would otherwise go right to your teeth.

COLLECTIBLES

How many of us keep business cards, restaurant mementos, corks, wine labels, etc.? But one never knows what to do with these things.

Buy a bolt of leather, and affix it to the top of a wall (appropriately in a den or an office). Place it so that you can pull down the leather and glue on, tape on, or pin on memorabilia.

One can also get a cabinetmaker to build a glass-front cabinet which will hold this while displaying your memories dust-free. Many stores have glass-front cabinets which would also do the trick.

The bolt allows the display of memories as you pull down more leather when needed.

NAIL FUNGUS
Fingers and Toes; Cuticle Infection

After trying every conceivable aid, I found that two products work!

1. **Peroxide**
   -Three percent hydrogen peroxide from the drugstore.
   -Sometimes as little as thirty-three cents for sixteen ounces when on sale.
   -Transfer some from the larger bottle to a small container (e.g., a clean old vitamin bottle).

-Use a small spoon every morning and also before bedtime for putting the peroxide under the affected nail; use enough to saturate the fungus. One can also use a Q-tip in order to put the peroxide under and around the nail. Be sure it is dry before putting on socks or hose. **You can use a blow dryer to hurry it along.**

2. **Grapefruit Seed Extract by NutriBiotic** (GSE)(I buy this from The Vitamin Shoppe in the two-ounce size, and the bottle has its own affixed top that sends out the extract drop by drop. The four-ounce size is too big). It is antifungal, antibacterial, antimicrobial.
-After showering at night (or just at bedtime), put a drop or two on tip of a small spoon (I use a plastic spoon) and dab it under and over the affected nail (use mini plastic disposable spoons). GSE will soak through the nail.
-It is strong and highly concentrated, and if you do this before going out as opposed to going to bed, it is necessary to give it time to dry before putting on hose. If you are going to put on hose and shoes, tuck a tiny piece of cotton under the toenail. I save cotton from vitamin bottles; I have not bought balls of cotton in many years! **I suggest, though, that one uses grapefruit seed extract before bed** rather than before going out and not risk getting this on your hose or on the inside of a shoe.
-I once got an **infection** under my **fingernail near the cuticle**. I put a drop of GSE onto the top of the nail (even over nail polish), and it soaked through and cleared up the infection in about three weeks.

Depending upon the depth of the fungus, it could take months to make headway (some people have had under-toenail fungus for years); however, these two products work! One can alternate weeks using these two products: one week for peroxide, one week for grapefruit seed extract.

After some weeks go by (possibly even longer), you will be surprised. Diligence is rewarded. Suddenly, after a shower, using the point of a nail file or small scissors, you will find that you can dislodge clumps and clumps of what <u>had</u> been affixed under your nail. It is now <u>dead</u> and is removable. Fungus is stubborn. It needs long treatment to beat it. I believe that it is pointless to take dangerous pills for a fungus at an extremity of the body when the sensible thing to do is go right to the extremity!

PROTECTING PANTYHOSE

From boots

The bane of our existence for those of us wearing stockings is snagged or runned pantyhose. Equally annoying are boots that snag the hose.

Solution: Take those pantyhose that are no longer wearable and cut each leg off at the upper thigh, and use these cutoff hose to pull over good hose when wearing boots.

For low boots, cut the legs at a lower point and roll gently just to the edge of the boot.

One winter night, I arrived at a favorite restaurant. As I sat outside the coat check, a woman patron watched me as I removed my boots, rolled off the protective hose from over my good hose, and put on my high heels. She said, "Wow! What a great idea! How did you ever think of that? I'm going to do that. You should write an advice column."

From toenails

The large toenail can be especially hard on hose. Tuck absorbent cotton around the nail tip and under the edge of the nail; then put on hose. Cotton cushions and protects the hose.

ABSORBENT COTTON

Cotton is used to stuff vitamin bottles and numerous other product bottles. Keep it, especially for removing nail polish as well as for tucking around toenails. I have not bought cotton balls in years.

HOW TO BRUSH ONE'S TEETH

Do you **know how** to brush the teeth? Angle the brush forty-five degrees with the bristles into the gums and between the teeth. **Wiggle** the brush between teeth as you work your way around, front and back. Do **not** abrade the gums and enamel by scrubbing. That will take a toll on the teeth over the years.

Do **not** look in the mirror while brushing because that will make you rush. Turn your back to the mirror. **Close your eyes**. Now give attention to all sides of your teeth. It should take two to three minutes if you brush properly.

Do see *Mybyble* article on Good-Gums. This is the product that I use for brushing my teeth. It allows the teeth to remineralize.

TOOTHBRUSHES, COLDS, BACTERIA, VIRUSES

Protecting ourselves from germs is a mighty task. We know about washing hands (including under the nails) for at least thirty seconds and not touching anything unnecessarily in public.

One easy habit is to use 3 percent hydrogen peroxide (standard drugstore item), and soak the toothbrush in it for five minutes once a week.

One can also soak brushes in household bleach once a week for five minutes, and then rinse with soapy water. Either product will produce a germ-free brush.

Always air-dry. I like to put our toothbrushes on a clean towel near sunlight from a window in order to let them dry with the added healthy boost of sunlight.

Washcloths: Always allow to air-dry *fully open*. Do **not** fold wet cloths in half! Bacteria thrive.

GOOD-GUMS FOR HEALTHY BRUSHING OF TEETH
Use Celtic Sea Salt in Water to Flush the Mouth All Day Long

I always have read that most toothpastes are useless in contributing to the health of the teeth and are dangerous as well (notice that some labels warn people **not** to swallow[!], and if a child or anyone swallows what covers the toothbrush, to immediately "call poison control"). Primarily, this is because most toothpastes have chemical ingredients as well as fluoride (not good—one never wants to swallow toxic substances) and *glycerin (which coats the teeth and prevents saliva from remineralizing them as nature intended!)*.

One day I am reading my "Health Sciences Institute" subscription newsletter (January 2012, vol. 16, no. 7), and there is the article on Good-Gums. I finally found this **all-natural powder—minus any chemicals—and** *safe even if some is swallowed*. I was especially impressed because it **contains grey sea salt** which, as I know, safely cleans teeth, refreshes breath, and improves gum health.

Good-Gums mixes with one's saliva (which is **full of healing enzymes** as you have read in *Mybyble*), and you then brush the moistened powder around teeth and gums (as instructed in article "How to Brush One's Teeth"). You can also dab Good-Gums on **sore spots**, and you can floss with the dissolved, saliva-liquefied powder. Do read the article on PULLING. Pulling Good-Gums through the teeth produces significant healing as well as nourishment. The benefits are legion.

<u>**SEA SALT**</u>: I searched for a long time before I found **Selina Naturally**. This is where I purchase what I consider to be one of the greatest sea salts: both the **(chunky) Light Grey Celtic Sea Salt** and the **(fine) Celtic Sea Salt**. I dissolve a teaspoon of chunky grey in a mug of pure room temperature water and use it all day every day for flushing my mouth after eating. The chunky grey contains the greatest percentage of healing minerals versus the fine (teaspoon versus teaspoon).

One can certainly also **gargle** with this and do **pulling** (see article "Pulling").

Personal Note: Good-Gums has absolutely made my mouth and that of others to whom I introduced it healthier. It heals gums by reducing or eliminating inflammation. Combining Good-Gums with GUM PerioBalance (see article "PROBIOTICS FOR GUMS AND PERIODONTAL DISEASE"), which is a *strain-specific* probiotic for the mouth, one can significantly improve mouth health.

If you add Selina Naturally Celtic Sea Salt water for swooshing the mouth to this daily protocol, the health benefits are astounding. And remember, all three products are **safe when** (or if) **swallowed! That says it all.**

See "Source List" for websites and telephones.

CELTIC SEA SALT WITH FOOD; GOOD SALT CRITICAL FOR GOOD HEALTH

Mental fog and brain issues can be symptoms of a deficiency!

In reference to Selina Naturally mentioned in the previous article, naturally, one should **always use this salt for foods** and never unhealthy, toxic refined sodium chloride table salt. **Celtic Sea Salt contains the natural minerals** that are so important to the body and balance our systems. It helps the **sinuses** (relieves mucus), nourishes the **adrenals** (which run on sodium [meaning Celtic Sea Salt sodium and not table salt]), **prevents illness** (by stimulating cellular energy and resistance in part due to its support of the adrenal glands), **can support normal blood pressure** (it is the bad salt that causes high blood pressure, not natural Celtic Sea Salt), contains **nutrients vital to the digestive system** and **helps the body digest food**, and does many other good, supportive things for the body.

Selina Naturally carries a vast line of healthful salts and other fine products. Keep natural products in mind when giving gifts.

Use Celtic Sea Salt on your various foods, and enjoy the enhanced taste from this natural, health supporting, nourishing product. REMEMBER: good salt is very important for health! **One symptom of a deficiency is a mental fog**. Sea salt is critical for brain and mental health. If you are having memory problems and other issues, use Celtic Sea Salt, and see if the issue was just a **symptom** of a deficiency of this nutrient.

FLOSS with FLOSS STICKS

I ignored flossing for years. I had no health issues with my mouth and could never get the hang of yanking floss through my teeth. One day someone introduced floss sticks to me. What an interesting product! It is a small plastic stick that is curved at one end with a piece of floss (shorter than three quarters of an inch) held taut in the curve.

I actually tried it that night after doing my teeth with Good-Gums. What a shock! There were still tiny particles in my gums that all my swooshing and rinsing had not dislodged. During the following several days, I tried the floss sticks many times after every meal and always found particles despite having rinsed with Celtic Sea Salt water.

While investigating several styles of floss sticks, I settled on Plackers Gentle Fine (for tight teeth) dental floss which I buy from Walgreens. I like the size and shape of the implement as well as the smoothness of the floss.

I carry a very small plastic seal-top bag in my purse in which I carry some extra floss sticks (as well as a Q-tip, a small emery board, and a couple of toothpicks) for emergencies.

Personal Note: For anyone who has ever broken a wrist—as I did just as I was completing proofreading my edited manuscript—one certainly knows that using regular floss is impossible when only one hand is functional. Floss sticks really come to the rescue in such a grievous situation.

PEROXIDE
Teeth, Gums, Sore Throat, Moles, Fungus

Three percent hydrogen peroxide is one of those amazing products. It is available, cheap, safe, and it works!

Teeth and Gums

Put a small amount of baking soda on the toothbrush. Dab the baking soda around the teeth. Then put three quarters of a teaspoon of peroxide into your mouth. Swoosh as it fizzes and foams. Then brush (per *Mybyble* article "How to Brush One's Teeth").

The wiggling bristles of a soft toothbrush will dislodge particles as will the fizzing peroxide. Even doing this twice a week—in addition to Good-Gums—is valuable.

Sore Throat

Put three quarters of a teaspoon of peroxide into three quarters of a cup of pure water. Gargle.

Moles

Certain moles will dry up and wash off with peroxide treatment. Use a Q-tip (or a toothpick or a plastic implement; for example, the back end of an eyeliner brush). Dip it into the peroxide (which you have transferred into a small container so as not to contaminate the larger bottle), and let the peroxide drip from it onto the mole. Do this morning and night.

Fungus

Under-the-toenail fungus is one of the most difficult types with which to deal. See *Mybyble* article "Nail Fungus".

CHOPSTICKS? NO! FUTURE STICKS!

I was recently introduced to a product that is just terrific. The founder of Future Sticks (who is from Texas) is married to a Chinese woman, and her mother has had severe arthritis for ten years which prohibits her from using her chopsticks. He adores his mother-in-law, and several years ago, he told his wife that he was working on **a new chopstick** (the original chopsticks were developed five thousand years ago) that **could be used not only by everyone who is healthy but also by folks with arthritis and Parkinson's.**

Even the most experienced chopstick user can experience difficulty in eating certain dishes. **Future Sticks offers a new patented feature on the chopstick: tiny teeth that increase the gripping power of the chopstick, making it possible for everyone to enjoy using chopsticks with ease and confidence.**

Future Sticks are made of a plastic polymer (called ULTEM, a SABIC, USFDA-certified food-grade plastic), and they do not release bisphenol A (BPA) gas when heated. They are **virtually unbreakable, dishwasher-safe**, and have the durability to be sterilized in an autoclave. This innovation creates a product that is sterile, reusable, portable, and capable of being carried to restaurants.

It is **ecofriendly** in that it **eliminates the need for disposable chopsticks** which use up natural resources. In China and Japan, this waste **claims more than 25 million full-grown trees each year.**

They also help with **personal health** because Future Sticks do not contain the mold or bleach that many disposable chopsticks do. This mold or bleach can leach into food while eating with the disposables. Future Sticks also help stop germs from being transmitted from person to person as is possible with reusable chopsticks.

With Future Sticks, experienced chopstick users can pick up the most difficult food with ease, while people with little experience using chopsticks can now eat without embarrassment. **Children love them**. It gives them confidence because they are fun while being functional. View the product and the unique story at www.futuresticks.com.

People with arthritis in their hands or with hand tremors (such as people with Parkinson's) can once again enjoy eating with chopsticks. The Future Stick design requires much less hand pressure, and the food resists being shaken off the chopstick.

Future Sticks are also a wonderful and unique gift, and they are **made in the USA. See "Source List" for a discount code.**

SKIN
Moisturize, Freshen

Keep either pure water (no fluoride or chlorine) or distilled* water in an atomizer to spray on the face in several ways:

1. After washing, spray the face in order to restore balance which soap and fluoridated water destroy.
2. Spray after makeup is complete in order to set it.
3. Spray while on airplanes to keep moist.
4. Spray in the office in order to remain fresh, especially if it is an office building with no open windows. Recirculated air removes moisture and is hard on the skin and also the mucous membranes in the nose. Everything gets dry.
5. Spray on hair in order to reblow it (anytime that your hair needs redoing).

*The reason that I mention distilled water for this use is because it is not congested with inorganic minerals. Thus, it can fully penetrate the skin and hair and truly be of benefit.

MOISTURIZE

Men and Women

Young, old, and in between, our skin needs attention. It does not, however, require expensive products to look its best. **What goes into the body is as important as what goes onto the body.** I avoid chemicals!

Women have asked me for years, "What do you use on your beautiful skin?" Here it is.

DRINK

In this case, pure water (both to drink and to spray on skin) is vital. By *pure* I mean without fluoride and chlorine as well as other toxic contaminants. Generally, one should drink—per day—two ounces for every pound of weight. Water is crucial for flushing your organs, and the skin is the largest organ. Water also suppresses hunger and saves the kidneys and liver from chronic overwork. When the kidneys are taxed from too little water, the **liver must take over**. Since the liver is your **number one fat-burning organ**, do you really want it processing liquids and toxins rather than BURNING FAT?

I will mention here that aside from regular bottled spring water, there is also distilled water. In the *Mybyble* article on spot cleaning, I indicate **why** distilled water is the **only** water to use. There are also times when drinking distilled water can be helpful. If one's system is congested, drinking distilled water for an entire day can help remove impurities. From time to time, I have used distilled water for one week or more in order to cleanse/remove inorganic residue which has been deposited in my system primarily from tap water.

To see just how pure spring and distilled water are, do a test. Take distilled, spring, and tap water. Pour each (in a separate line) down the (clean) side of a car. Only the distilled leaves no spots or streaks. The spring water follows, but it depends upon what brand of water and from which springs the water originated. There are some springs that are shallow, and the water bottled from those springs is not as pure or sediment-free as that which is bottled from deep springs. It is the same inside your body. Pure water would leave little to no contaminants versus those waters that leave inorganic residue.

Beware of buying bottled water that is actually municipal water. READ those labels!

Regarding drinking distilled water occasionally, anyone who says that distilled water leaches out minerals while other waters provide minerals is somewhat misadvised. One: if we relied upon water for nutrients, we would be dead. Two: other waters leave inorganic, unusable minerals rather than organic, useful minerals. Three: distilled water does not deplete our body of nutrients inasmuch as it can help remove that built-up residue clogging every areaway of our bodies.

SPRAY

Keep distilled or spring water in a small atomizer to spray on the skin both before and after applying makeup. It sets the makeup. Drink and spray on airplanes and in offices.

CREAM/OIL

On young skin, a mild cream or lotion suffices. But as we age and skin is not as plump and moist, more is needed, and for all ages, a moisturizer must be pure. It must **help** the skin and not burden it. By *burden*, I mean not clogging the pores or having chemicals in it or useless ingredients. Just because a product is pricey does not mean that it is the best product out there. In fact, some of the best skin products cost very little.

There are four important oils. One must be aware, though, that all oils are not equal. There are certain oils that tend to *not* clog pores, and they are, therefore, noncomedogenic in nature. They allow pores to function and breathe.

Some of these oils—which I use—are Omega Nutrition Organic Virgin Coconut Oil, Thunder Ridge Emu Oil, Mayumi Squalane, and Desert Essence Organic Jojoba Oil. The first two I buy direct from the producers, and the second two I buy from either The Vitamin Shoppe, Swanson, or Vitacost. These three suppliers have varied sales during the year as well (See "Source List"). (*See article* "Face and Neck Moisturizers: Skin Care" for complete information.)

NIGHT

At night after washing (see *Mybyble* article "Face and Neck Moisturizers: Skin Care" which explains using coconut oil to remove makeup and wash the face rather than soap), I generally use emu oil all over my face and neck. On the neck, make sure to also pat the **emu oil on and below the Adam's apple where the thyroid gland is located** (just below the Adam's apple approximately where a bow tie would sit). Emu oil sinks deeply into the skin, and in this particular spot, it will nourish the important thyroid.

Organic virgin coconut oil can also be used exactly the same way. After using it to remove all makeup, it can then be patted onto the face, neck, and over the thyroid gland. It, too, penetrates deeply and beneficially into the skin.

DAY

For daytime, spray the face with distilled or spring water in order to hydrate as well as normalize the pH if any tap water was used. When I am short of time, that is one step that I eliminate, especially since my face has been moisturized the night before with either emu or coconut oil.

Lightly dab squalane around the eyes and mouth and use jojoba on the cheeks and chin. These two oils are not greasy but sink into the skin while leaving the sheerest moisture for under makeup. The forehead should not receive oil as it is usually more oily than the rest of the face. Additionally, one does not want oil to get into the hairline.

For additionally moisturized skin prior to putting on makeup, one can use Nivea Creme patted on after the jojoba oil. I use Nivea Creme between the eyebrows and on the cheeks, chin, and upper lip. I like to have a glistening look to my skin as well as having makeup look luscious. Makeup goes on beautifully, and your skin has a lustrous glow. One point of information: Nivea Creme deviates from all the other products that I mentioned. It has chemicals and other ingredients in it. I do not use it daily, and I would never use it unless I first had squalane and jojoba oil as the base. Most people will find these two oils to be a sufficient moisturizing base for applying makeup.

From the products mentioned, it is clear that they are not high-priced designer products. There *are* high-priced products which have actually used emu oil and coconut oil as ingredients. I believe in reducing or eliminating all the additives and chemicals and using only the purest products.

Personal Note: I was twenty years old and was at a dinner party. The hostess was a very wealthy lady of forty-five years of age. Her skin was glowing, and I asked her what products she used. She put her arm around me, chuckled, and said, "Carole, let me tell you that everyone thinks surely I buy these crazy, expensive creams and makeup. Forget it! I use Nivea Creme for everything. You should try it. I buy it at the drugstore." That was my introduction to Nivea. I buy it at CVS.

MEN

Men are taking more care of their skin nowadays. Coconut oil and emu oil are excellent at night or for days at home. The oils penetrate many layers into the skin and promote healthy complexions.

Emu oil is also used in a **shaving product** from Thunder Ridge. I have given it as a gift to some men, and they thought it was terrific. I know another gentleman who uses the coconut oil for shaving.

MAKEUP BASE

Many women ask me about my makeup foundation. Therefore, I am including this because I do not use a typical liquid foundation. I just love what I have used since around my late twenties.

I like a creamy finish. The easiest base to use for this effect is Elizabeth Arden's Flawless Finish pressed cream compact. Elizabeth Arden has never changed the product, and that consistency is a joy.

I use two shades (porcelain beige and warm beige). Warm beige (just a speck darker) is good for the nose and chin, while I use the softer porcelain beige everywhere else.

The compact comes with a sponge placed in a small compartment in front of the makeup. This compartment has a vented (bunch of tiny holes) bottom in order to allow the sponge to dry. I detest the sponge as well as the holes. First, by using clean fingertips, you get much better control and finish as well as not wasting a huge amount of makeup on the sponge. Get rid of the sponge, or use it for something else. Secondly, get a roll of adhesive tape, and from the <u>inside</u> of the compact, cover the holes. These holes let in dust and minute particles. Seal them up, and have a nice, clean compact!

Once you use up the makeup in one of the compacts, use it in your purse for carrying small amounts of both foundations. I use a tiny spatula (which came with some other makeup long ago; it is about two inches long, and the tiny spatula end is about a quarter inch wide [one can also use the point of a very small knife]), and I gently scrape a small amount of porcelain beige and put that on one side of the now-empty compact; then I collect some warm beige and put it on the other side of the compact. It is perfect for touching up my nose or chin during a long business day.

CREAM EYE SHADOW and CHEEK BLUSH (ROUGE)

It is often difficult to find that **exact (absolutely precise)** color that one wants in a **cream** eye shadow or rouge (blush) as well as to find the perfect creamy texture. I **use lipstick!** It is so easy to gently stroke the color on eyelids or, for cheeks, dab a bit of color on a finger and pat it on the cheek. I prefer cream over powder because it does not cake, allows me to stroke or pat on a sheer veneer, and gives me more control (than powder).

I prefer a soft, shimmery silver on my eyelids. It goes with everything and looks nice on me. I used to exclusively buy Wet n' Wild until the company was sold and the products were changed. Heartbreak! But yes, they are still available (in fewer colors) if you check several drugstores for inventory of the color for which you are searching. I have also found a myriad of colors and textures in the Sephora Collection *in the store* www.sephora.com. Online I do not see all the colors. They are reasonably priced for a makeup boutique.

Of course, **how can one beat CVS or Walgreens for Wet n' Wild, Revlon, Maybelline,** and **Rimmel (plus others)**? There is a total selection, one can certainly find a color for the eyelid or cheeks, and opened products are returnable! What better customer service could one want?

Personal Note: You will join me in a good laugh at this *note*. When I was growing up, my mother purchased name cosmetics in elegant department stores. She taught me to buy fine manufacturers. One had one's salesgirl (usually an older lady) for years! She took care of you, and you were loyal to her!

When I was around thirty, I was at a formal dinner and admired the lipstick on a woman and asked what color it was. She opened a $900 minaudière (elegant small evening bag) to "pop" out a 99¢ (at that time [and not much more now]) Wet n' Wild lipstick! Oh, did we laugh. A $900 bag with a 99¢ lipstick. I remember still today her chortling, "I seem to have brought out all the '9s' tonight."

But that was typical. Elegant, expensively dressed women got a kick out of this "show". There were two products that were (and are) cheap and irreplaceable: **Wet n' Wild** lipstick (and nail polish) and **Maybelline Great Lash Mascara (**for me **in royal blue**—the only mascara that I have ever used!).

More to this Personal Note: At one time, I met the public relations director of one of the most expensive cosmetics companies of that time. He and I got quite chummy as we compared notes on various cosmetics. Then I told him the Wet n' Wild lipstick story. He cracked up! Then he became serious and lowered his voice and said, "If I tell you something, will you hold it in complete confidence? If this ever got out, I would lose my job." Of course, I promised total secrecy. "Well," he murmured, "I want you to know that some of *our* most popular lipstick colors are available through Wet n' Wild with different names for those colors, of course. Ninety-nine cents a tube instead of twenty dollars." Was I ever taken aback! I then realized that it is not just spending crazy amounts of money for a product, but it is also *knowing* what you are buying. I always knew that some less costly products were good *quality*. It is certainly true today. Try a lipstick for your eyelids and cheeks. Why not?

BUFFING SKIN OR FACE

The skin is continuously sloughing off dead cells; however, it needs help getting rid of this debris. Since the skin is delicate, handle this tenderly.

First, remove makeup with coconut oil as described in *Mybyble* article "Washing the Face, Removing Makeup".

Once or twice a week is sufficient for buffing facial skin (although when one showers, it is always good to use a loofah from the chest to the toes). The easiest, cheapest, and best method for helping the face exfoliate is soap and warm water. Use a nice, *soft*, washcloth (100 percent Egyptian cotton is very soft and is often on sale at T.J. Maxx and sometimes at JCPenney). Soap it up as well as the face.

Tip: Using the soapy washcloth: **use it in circular motions all over the face. To be sure that your touch is gentle, use counterclockwise motions and use your <u>non</u>dominant hand! These two things will keep your touch light.** Should the face be suffering from any irritation, do not buff it. Stay with using the virgin coconut oil.

Towel

Use a soft linen towel for drying the face and ears while gently buffing the skin to help it exfoliate. Again, do not buff if there is any existing facial irritation.

Soap

Liquid natural soap (concentrated) from Omega Nutrition is good on a loofah. Alternatively, one can use a glycerin soap from Puritan's Pride (three for one and other sales several times yearly) which gives a really nice lather.

NOTE: If there is any rash or irritation, one should not buff. Use coconut oil to wash the face *very gently;* do not agitate any irritation. See "Face and Neck Moisturizers".

STOCKINGS, PANTYHOSE, VARICOSE VEINS, SPIDER VEINS
Support for Impaired Circulation

In order to enhance the appearance of the leg, wear one pair of pantyhose; and if needed, wear <u>two</u> pair! I really cannot understand females going bare-legged when they have scrawny, bony, blotchy, veiny, and otherwise unattractive legs or flabby thighs. Just look in the mirror! One watches television and sees these stars cross their imperfect legs and wonders, *Just how big an ego do you have to display those bony knees or legs [thinking that they are great] or mottled thighs rather than sheathing them in stunning hose?*

One pair of pantyhose is perfect for most legs as well as supplying mild or stronger support if circulation is impaired. There are so many strengths available today, including sheer, regular, sheer support, medium support, and others. Additionally, pantyhose in nasty or cold weather are wonderful. There are also stunning tights which enhance the look of any outfit.

Using a nice taupe or suntan shade as the underneath color, one can enhance dark shades or pale shades. I like taupe under black, off black, burgundy, and other dark colors. I like suntan under pale green, pale gray, or other pale shades.

The double hose choice gives the leg a silky, satiny look, camouflages slight to serious flaws, and is especially warming in cold weather.

In warm weather, the double hose is best in air-conditioned environments; however, it does give a nice tan look to the leg (for example, a suntan shade under a deeper suntan shade). Considering the aggravation of **spider veins** and heavier **varicose veins**, this is a cosmetic solution at all times of the year.

Pantyhose under fishnets also are a much more attractive, finished look than bare skin.

During **pregnancy**, one might appreciate extra support for the legs and for circulation but cannot have pantyhose around the waist. Thigh-high hose will suffice and are available in various support strengths. There are also knee-high hose which some find useful.

PERFUME OR MEN'S COLOGNE OR AFTERSHAVE
Use PETROLEUM JELLY (Vaseline or House Brand)

Use a <u>sheer</u> dab of petroleum jelly on wrists and behind the ears. Put your perfume or cologne <u>over</u> it. The fragrance will last much longer than when put only on the skin.

Personal Note: I love this tip so much that I included it twice. It is also in "Tips, Tips, and More Tips!" A marvelous scent enhances any woman or man's persona.

CAMOUFLAGE FLAWS

Makeup counters would like to sell you the most expensive items for camouflaging under-eye circles or darkness and also spider veins on the legs.

For 73¢ to $2.00 (depending upon the sale), one can buy Wet n' Wild (at CVS, Walgreens, and others) cover stick concealer (it looks like a lipstick) in 801 light (or medium 804). For the legs, rub it over the defect, pat with a finger, and put on your hose.

For under-eye camouflage, you need a soft tiny brush. (See *Mybyble* on "Eye Makeup Brushes"). Run it over the 801 light, and then stroke or dab the tiny brush on the dark area under the eye. Dot the concealer *only on the dark rim* of the circle under the eye. Pat with finger.

Remember, when you use up the part of the concealer stick that shows (similar to a lipstick), there is a large amount of product beneath the rim; this is perfect to save for eye repairs. Additionally, you can scrape out small layers with the back end of tweezers or a tiny spatula and pat onto leg spider veins with your fingers. No need to throw it away.

Of course, one must do the under-eye camouflage over well-moisturized skin. Please read article "Face and Neck Moisturizers". Sheer moisture allows easier use of 801 light and prevents it from caking.

Women and Men: Camouflage nose pores: Certainly women would use this tip, but I also know men who wish to cover pores in the nose. Any creamy liquid makeup base that is exactly one's skin tone can be rubbed into the nose pores in order to camouflage them. The makeup is unobtrusive and conceals those oversized pores.

EYELID IRRITATION

Once in a while, especially due to the use of makeup or getting a germy finger near the eye, one gets irritation/itching along the eyelashes. It is usually along the lower lashes and toward the inner corner of the eye or the upper lashes toward the inner corner.

Sometimes, a quick **spray of spring or distilled water** (from an atomizer) will stop the burning or itching.

Alternatively, I keep **George's Always Active® Aloe Vera** (which I buy from Vitacost) on hand and transfer it from the 128 ounce bottle to a very small bottle (for example, an old vitamin bottle that is carefully washed). Use a Q-tip and dab it into the aloe water. Run the Q-tip along the eyelid that is itchy. This usually helps very quickly. Remember that one can also drink this aloe vera water. It tastes just like spring water and is used for digestion. It contains no preservatives or additives.

Another soothing treatment is **emu oil** which is mentioned in several *Mybyble* articles. Dot a little emu onto a Q-tip and run that along the irritated eyelid. This is quite calming.

One's **urine** can also be effective. See the article on *urine*. Again, dab a Q-tip into one's own urine (leaving it just barely wet), and stroke it onto the irritated area.

Should the first treatment not cure the irritation, one can repeat any of these treatments a few times a day. It should also get rid of any pending infection by opening the pores or eyelash follicles and cleaning whatever is there that is causing the itch or irritation. I find that if I use, for example, water, aloe, or urine first and that does not immediately get rid of the irritation, I promptly go to emu oil.

Which treatment is effective depends upon what caused the itching or irritation. One of these several solutions should usually work. Should any of these products accidentally get into the eye, they are not harmful. Just use a tissue to dab it out.

HEAT—OR COLD—TREATMENT
Injuries, Muscle Pain, Joint Pain

If you injure a hand or finger for which heat is the prescribed treatment, it is very soothing to pull on a fleece-lined rubber glove and hold your hand under hot running water. Depending upon the injury, one can even use the bathtub and run the tap for stronger pressure.

For a foot or lower leg that needs this treatment, pull on a rubber boot (similar to a fisherman's wader), sit on the edge of the bathtub, read something or listen to the radio or television, and let the tub water run over the boot.

Conversely, if cold is prescribed, use cold water.

If there is an injury needing warmth for treatment, one can also use a hair blower. As long as one's arm can get the blower positioned to blow warm air on the injured area, this can be a quickly soothing solution. I use a travel-sized blower because the low wattage sends out a more gentle air flow.

EAR PRESSURE, AIRPLANES

If you need to yawn in order to pop your ears on an airplane, entwine your fingers (one hand's fingers grabbing the other hand's fingers) and pull, keeping your chest high and elbows out (not dropped). The energy paths thus created cause one to yawn.

Also, with elbows out and hands chest-high, press palms (fingers upward) firmly together to count of ten. Repeat. Sometimes this pressing rather than pulling causes a yawn more quickly.

Both of these exercises are **isometrics**. Remember to **pull or press and create tension.**

EYE MAKEUP

Applying mascara perfectly can be tricky. I keep a hat pin (a straight pin longer than a regular pin and with a little knob at one end) as well as a toothpick at hand. The pin (used <u>*cautiously*</u>) can separate any clumps. The toothpick, run along beneath lower lashes, can remove any smudges.

Also, when one gets fuzz or similar from a hat, coat, or sweater caught in the eyelashes, if you slowly and carefully run a toothpick along the lower or upper lid, it will catch the offending matter while not ruining eye makeup.

SLEEP FACTS and SLEEPING POSITIONS:
Face Wrinkles, Backache, Circulation, Venous Insufficiency

Our body's most recuperative time is during sleep. Maximizing those hours is critical.

Position is important, since such a major amount of time over our lifetimes is spent sleeping. The preferred position is on one's back. This is best for preventing facial wrinkles (not smooshing one's face into a pillow night after night) by letting one's face relax and allowing gravity to act *for* you instead of against. By sleeping on the back, gravity is pulling the face into its smoothest position. **Take a mirror, lie down on your back, and look at your face versus standing up or lying on your side or, even worse, face into the pillow. See? When on your back, your face looks youthful.**

If you do lie on your side, it is better to lie on your right side—away from the heart. Scrunching any vital organs is not to your advantage. Lying on the back allows organs their maximum position of relief. They can, so to speak, spread out.

Personal Note: Over the years while dining at fine Manhattan restaurants, we have met a delightful gentleman and enjoyed conversation together. The September 29, 2013 issue of *The New York Times* offered a wonderful interview with this **_103(!)-year-old man_**. He comments, "I read in a newspaper column a long time ago that **the key to a long life is sleeping on your back**, so I always did that." I salute Mr. Harry Rosen and wish him continued years of dining pleasure as well as good health from sleeping on his back.

In order to relieve lower-back tension and certain other problems such as circulation, there are two places under which to place a pillow. To **take pressure off the back**, place a medium-volume pillow under the upper thighs just below the buttocks. One can test which pillow fullness provides relief: a flatter pillow or a medium-volume one. For **circulatory problems**, I had mild **venous insufficiency** in my left leg. I found that putting a pillow under my right ankle while placing my left leg slightly off to the left side of the pillow (and flat on the mattress) worked best for me. You need to try several positions with the pillow depending upon what is causing your circulatory problems.

It is also very beneficial to **"shake your organs" into proper place before sleep**. Lying on your back, with head on the pillow, have arms flat on the bed next to your body with palms on the mattress, bend your knees with feet flat on the mattress, and elevate your pelvis. Giggle/wiggle a bit, allowing organs to get into proper place while you sleep. Close your eyes when doing this. It focuses you. See article "Close Your Eyes".

After you giggle/wiggle and you are lying flat again, point the toes of one foot and extend that leg forward while pulling back the hip of the other side. Then do the other foot and hip. This, too, helps the **spine, the hip area, and the general body alignment** before sleep (or any time of the day). For extra emphasis, when you point the toes, gently *lift* that leg a couple of inches while extending it forward and pulling the opposite hip backward. I do just one or two before sleep, and as always, I close my eyes in order to visualize the movement.

Remember that for the kidneys, 11:00 pm to 1:00 am is when they go into action performing their functions while one sleeps, and from 1:00 am to 3:00 am, the liver is functioning. If you never get to sleep by 11:00 pm, your kidneys and liver are stymied in their repair functions. Every organ of the body has repair/maintenance time throughout the twenty-four-hour cycle, but **maintenance during our sleeping time is critical.** *Have you ever noticed that you went to bed with a bad pimple or a pain somewhere or a strain, and when you awakened, the problem was either all better or less severe?* **Sleep time is healing time.**

TOTAL DARKNESS FOR SLEEPING: Healthy sleeping depends upon melatonin production, and artificial light suppresses it. This indefatigable biochemical is produced by the brain's pineal gland *in darkness* and regulates our sleep/wake cycle. It lowers blood pressure, glucose levels, and body temperature—key physiological responses which are responsible for restful sleep. Artificial light (as well as the electric blanket) disrupts sleep which, in turn, results in many health problems. So, say NO to a clock radio (put a towel over it), the monitor on an air-conditioner (cover it), and certainly to computer monitors or other screens with light in the bedroom (none of which should ever be in a bedroom!). Definitely use opaque curtains or drapes in order to eliminate outside light. For a restful sleep, one should avoid artificial light for at least one hour before bedtime. **HISTORY:** Before electricity, we had sunlight and, at night, moonlight, starlight, and campfire light. This was natural light which governed regulating the circadian rhythm. Every form of artificial light to which we are subjected today—particularly after sunset—interferes with our biological processes and elevates cortisol at night which disturbs sleep and creates other health problems.

Personal Note: Recently, the area where I reside suffered a power outage starting at 4:00 PM. We had absolutely no light from any source. I immediately lit candles. We had a small dinner by candlelight (my stove is gas, not electric), talked, and finally went to bed at 8:46 PM at which time I was really exhausted. The sun had set soon after the power went out, and we were now functioning on the caveman's lifestyle. I enjoyed the deepest sleep! Try this sometime at sunset, and experience real sleep due to light as nature meant it to be.

EYE MAKEUP BRUSHES

It becomes ever more difficult to <u>find</u> perfect quality sable eye makeup brushes at <u>reasonable</u> prices. For years I bought a brush from Max Factor. Alas, that disappeared from the shelves. I was nearly at a loss regarding finding a suitable brush when, some years back, I was travelling on business and walking in downtown Traverse City, Michigan. I found a superb art supply store and suddenly thought, *Maybe they sell small brushes!* That is where I found and bought Escoda brushes (*sable with an ultrafine tip,* excellent for putting on cake eyeliner) and Yasutomo brushes. There are also other styles suited to doing eye shadow and cheeks. This store closed down when the owner retired.

Currently, I buy Escoda brushes from Jerry's Artarama. I buy the *sable and synthetic* Yasutomo brush that has a *sturdier tip* directly from Yasutomo (see "Source List"). Both companies have sales throughout the year and are so very nice to speak with on the telephone or order online. As is so often the case, I find better prices <u>out</u> of the big cities (such as away from my home in New York).

The important point here is: use a good art supply store for makeup brushes.

TECHNIQUE FOR USING EYE CREAMS/ MOISTURIZING
Toning Skin around the Eyes

When patting cream or Mayumi Squalane around the eyes, *patting* is the key word. Gently pat the moisturizers, going from the inner corner out on the <u>upper</u> lid and from the outer corner in <u>beneath</u> the eyes. This path is the healthy path for skin around the eyes.

You <u>never</u> want to rub and stretch this extremely delicate tissue. Over the years, harsh treatment (even though you may not <u>think</u> you are doing harm) will take its toll.

A relaxing and wrinkle-easing exercise while you are lying down or inverted on your slant board is to pat around your eyes with the <u>pads</u> of your fingers. Go, as instructed, from the inner corner out (over the eyelid) and from the outer corner in beneath the eye.

Chinese medicine teaches about energy paths. This is one of them.

BOWEL, STOOL, ELIMINATION, CONSTIPATION, BABIES AND POTTIES, SUPPORT FOR BLADDER

People should optimally have a bowel movement three times daily (or even more). Just like a baby—eat and poop!

As we go through life, however, our habits alter. Incorrect diet, pressures of daily life, time constraints, all can inhibit regular movements. That is when some of these tips are so helpful. If the morning is *your* time, then before you get out of bed, turn onto your left side, and relax there. Lying on the left side can stimulate the bowel. Three to ten minutes could stimulate a movement.

1. Find the time of day that you really get the urge to go. For many people this is soon after arising and before or after having a cup of warm water. For others, it is once they have had some morning food (preferably, fruit). Peristalsis is triggered, and that pressures the bowel.
2. Do not ever ignore the urge. If you eat with people and cannot just leave the table, excuse yourself by saying that something got in your eye. Say anything, but go!
3. Find a place where you are comfortable going. If at business, do you have a choice of one toilet or another? Line the seat with extra tissue in order to make it easier on your tush. At home, just relax.
4. Position: Our toilets are horrendously designed for easing elimination. Optimally, **knees should be <u>above</u> the thighs.**

That is the perfect position. This position goes back to the days before there were toilets when people **squatted** in the fields or elsewhere in order to eliminate. This was the natural position. **Squatting straightens the rectum which facilitates elimination**, and the straightened anal canal relieves SO MANY bowel problems. Look at children! Babies automatically squat to defecate. That is the normal, functional position. Sitting on potties is not beneficial to pooping, and **babies having trouble with potties** have simply not yet transitioned from the natural habit of squatting to using a toilet. Squatting also allows immediate and complete evacuation (of stool), whereas some people sit forever on toilets (and read newspapers) while waiting. This is so unhealthy and leads to hemorrhoids and constipation, and the latter can lead to colorectal cancer. Hence, people in the know seek to buy Asian squat toilets, or, just toilets which are lower to the ground.

    NOTE REGARDING **THE <u>BLADDER:</u>** Proper elimination supports the bladder (with an improved pelvic floor nerve supply) and can, in time, improve bladder function.

So, lacking a low commode at home, have a sturdy small wastebasket on which you can place your feet, or turn it on its side and place your feet on it. Today, in many restaurant bathrooms, small wastebaskets are placed near toilets. Use it for your feet! With feet up, one can also **tilt the pelvis up which straightens the rectum and hastens an easy elimination** (as I wrote before).

Barring that comfort, learn to raise your knees or extend your legs with feet pressed against the bathroom door in order to help the body eliminate easily.

Additionally, **here are some major tips for opening the body's elimination channels:**

1. Place your palms together, fingers pointed upward, elbows out at chest level; press the palms and hold to a count of ten. Release. Repeat. These isometrics ease the stool flow. It has to do with energy paths. Also, entwining fingers and *pulling* <u>really</u> opens the elimination channel! If you shut your eyes

and try to open the lids <u>without</u> doing so (while pulling your arms), you actually complete the opening and easing of the elimination channel. I learned this some years back from a Chinese doctor who discussed energy paths.

2. Which exercise works depends upon where the feces are within the system (how high up). Sometimes one needs to put both arms up in the air, grasp each elbow with the opposite hand, and twist the torso slightly to the right. That can also open the elimination pathway. Also, a slight variation: put arms up in the air and grasp hands. Raising the arms **lengthens the torso and helps straighten the anal canal and rectum** which can help elimination, especially if the feet are elevated either on a stepstool or are pressed straight against a closed door in front of you. **Tilting the pelvis slightly upward at the same time will also straighten the rectum and anal canal.** This supports a natural elimination!

3. If you are having a problem eliminating, bend over (as though reaching to pick something up on the floor) or squat. These two positions help move the bowel into position, and elimination should come. Sometimes one is standing up and feels the urge to go, and then when sitting on the toilet (in that unnatural position), the urge seems to disappear; in that case, bend forward. Place your chest to your knees. You just need to **move the stool downward and straighten the anal canal and rectum.**

4. You will also find that blowing air from your nose (simulate blowing the nose into a tissue) opens the elimination track. Although bowel movements should optimally be three times daily, many people find that they go several times at a particular time of day rather than spaced out. Two to five times during an entire morning is just as good as spaced out all day. Whatever works for you is fine! Just go.

5. **Water and fiber** are also so important. A cup of **warm pure water** upon arising (some folks enjoy it with raw organic honey and apple cider vinegar [see *Mybyble* article "Honey

and Apple Cider Vinegar"] while others prefer fresh lemon squeezed in) *can stimulate peristalsis*. Or a movement can be stimulated after eating **whole fresh fruit on that empty stomach**. Eating whole fruit first thing in the morning is the healthiest time and is the most nutritious for the body. See article "Food Combining".

Drink pure water all during the day as well as cups of warm water. Movements that are hard indicate a lack of moisture. Hydrate the body. **Another symptom of the body needing water is when the corners of the mouth seem to sweat.** You actually go to dab at the corners because they seem to be damp; however, there is nothing there. It is a symptom of dehydration. So is a hard stool. I mentioned this in "Tips!".

Vegetables before dinner provide necessary fiber which can help facilitate a late-evening movement or one the next morning. **Avoid artificial sweeteners, excess sugar (especially fructose), chemical additives, MSG, excessive amounts of caffeine, and processed foods as they are all detrimental to the gastrointestinal (and immune) function. Eat WHOLE foods, get exercise, hydrate with pure water, and avoid pharmaceutical drugs** (painkillers like codeine or hydrocodone can **slow bowel function**, while antidepressants and antibiotics can also **cause a variety of GI disruptions**; read drug information sheets for contraindications / side effects).

Do refer to *Mybyble* article on "Coconut or Emu Oil for Derrières (Buttock, Anal, and Rectal Distress)" and for wiping tips!

SALIVA, NAIL POLISH

When you are polishing your nails and nick or smudge it, if you are in a rush, you can gently lick it with your tongue. Saliva will smooth the nick or smudge. If done at bedtime, it will dry as you sleep.

At first, the saliva-on-polish is slightly sticky until fully dry.

Chipping Nail Polish

If you chip your polish, put a dot of clear polish around the chip and smush around the spot with the nail polish brush. The clear polish liquefies the color polish which then runs into the chipped spot.

This is much more effective than just trying to fill in the chip with color which never leaves a smooth finish.

When the chip repair dries, you can then dab on the color polish (if even necessary).

SALIVA and URINE CONTAIN HEALING ENZYMES
Stop a Run in Stockings / Pantyhose with Saliva

People get a paper cut and promptly put the injured digit to the tongue. It is a reflex action, because saliva contains healing enzymes, and we see so many people do this all the time. In the case of a paper cut, though, one's urine will seal the cut more quickly and effectively than saliva.

Go to the bathroom, and either put your finger into the stream of urine or put urine on toilet tissue and wrap it around where the cut is. You only need to leave the urine there for a few seconds and then dab it dry. (See *Mybyble* article "Urine to the Rescue.")

Should you accidently bite the inside of your mouth or tongue or suddenly get a twinge in a tooth and you cannot get to the dentist, **run the tip of your tongue along the gum behind your lower teeth**. This will cause saliva to be produced which you can then swish onto the injured gum or tongue or around the tooth suffering a twinge. Do this for several minutes in order to calm the aggravated spot or to soothe the tooth until you see if that twinge returns. The healing enzymes in saliva can help in these situations.

If you wear pantyhose or stockings and you get a run, put a lot of saliva all over the run and especially at the end point. The enzymes in saliva can help halt the run.

HOT FLASHES

Breathe

Deep breaths (see *Mybyble* "Breathing" article) are an immediate, stabilizing, balancing influence on the body.

Take in breath <u>slowly</u> through the nose (as if blowing up a balloon in the stomach) and <u>*hold it*</u> for a few seconds before releasing. This helps reset the body. *It is <u>the best tip</u> I ever found regarding hot flashes*. The longer you gently hold the breath, the better, because it is working to stabilize your system! And, you can do this breathing anywhere.

Keep your *eyes closed* while doing this (see *Mybyble* articles "Close Your Eyes" and "Breathe") in order to focus on the soothing, steady breath coming in; hold that breath; let the body balance itself before you **expel** the breath **through the mouth**. Repeat.

Herbs and Legume

There are a couple of herbs, one legume, and one supplement that seem to address the hormone issues. Every woman's body is different, and since these supplements are nontoxic and not cumulative, one can try each.

Alfalfa: The best herbal medical tip for hot flashes that I ever read was for alfalfa which is rich in vitamins and minerals and **is actually a legume**, not an herb. It alkalizes the body and is a cooling, sweet, astringent legume that can help moderate hot flashes and night sweats. Alfalfa has deep roots which bring many nutrients into the plant and thus into the nutrient-rich end product.

Maca is a natural hormone balancer. For therapeutic use, it is important to purchase a maca powder that is organic, raw, and fresh. This gives the greatest chance of success. The dosage should be about one teaspoon per day in the beginning, working up to one to two tablespoons until one begins to feel the symptoms disappear. Stop at the lowest successful dose. No need to do more.

Maca powder (in water, has taste of malt) creates a large coated surface area which provides easier absorption by the intestines, thus getting the nutrients into the bloodstream and endocrine system faster than via tablet/capsule.

Vitex (chaste berry) is used to balance hormones and also to promote good sleep.

Bee Propolis (500 mg., four to six capsules daily) can be helpful. Additionally, using **raw organic honey and apple cider vinegar** (see *Mybyble* article) can also be a calmative.

Pumpkin seeds: Organic raw pumpkin seeds are loaded with nutrients, and numerous articles suggest pumpkin seeds for helping with hot flashes. Certainly it could not hurt!

FISH OIL for HEALTH (and Even Hot Flashes, Inflammation, Stroke Prevention)

The right fish oil can provide omega-3s which, for some women, will help alleviate hot flashes. It is crucially important, though, to use a fish oil that has *whole* omegas and provides full nutritional value. It was a long search before I found *New Chapter's Wholemega Whole Fish Oil*. It is that word *whole* that indicates that the soft gels contain the ingredients of the whole fish.

I like what I first read in their newsletter: "New Chapter is proud to offer a whole-food approach to fish oil and an alternative to the fractionated, highly processed, and high-heat purified oils on the market today" and "Wholemega is 100% wild-caught salmon oil that is naturally pure."

In other words—and critical—they do NOT fractionate or highly process their Wholemega Fish Oil, and the capsule contains 100 percent wild-caught salmon from protected Alaskan waters as opposed to an amalgamation of fish caught heaven knows where and combined into a capsule. The Wholemega label indicates *all* the vitamins and nutrients actually in Wholemega. This is significant. Wholemega delivers the natural profile of seventeen omega fatty acids. Other product labels do not contain this information.

I buy the product from Swanson or Vitacost, and both companies offer regular sales. Go online to either company, pull up Wholemega, then click on Read Label (or it may just say Label). One is able to view the entire label as opposed to whatever product one is currently taking or to which one is comparing Wholemega! **When one takes fish oil, it should always be with some fats in the tummy** because *fish oil is fat soluble.* So many people recommend fish oil but never stress taking it when there are fats in the tummy, thus allowing the fish oil to be digested.

Omega fatty acids may help **reduce inflammation and risk of blood clot formation**. Plus, **these fatty acids may lower the chance of developing stroke risk factors, such as heart disease and high blood pressure.**

FISH OIL and VITAMIN A
Cracks on the Heels—Both on the Inner Side of the Heel and on the Outside of the Heel

The *right* fish oil provides many needed nutrients to the body and can offer both preventive and therapeutic support regarding certain conditions. One can read online about fish oil benefits. It has a high level of beneficial omega-3 fatty acids, and the *right* fish oil provides so much more. It has anti-inflammatory properties as well as positive effects on the composition of the body. When I first read this last advisement ("positive effects of the composition of the body"), it occurred to me that I might have found a cure for the cracks in my heels.

AMAZING Personal Note: I had developed *cracks on the inner side of my heels.* I searched at great length to find what deficiency was causing this until I read what I wrote above. I started taking what was reputed to be a fine, well-known fish oil. It seemed to help a little but was by no means a cure. Then I heard a radio commercial for New Chapter Wholemega (be sure to read the previous article), and I knew that I had the solution. I ordered the product, and within three days, the cracks on the inside of my heels were diminishing. Within ten days, they were gone. I thought to myself, *Just imagine what deficiencies inside your body are being eliminated!*

Now we come to **vitamin A**. While many supplements provide beta-carotene and say that the body will convert it into vitamin A as needed, the fact is that one may actually need to take a vitamin A supplement. Only a portion of beta-carotene is converted to vitamin A within the body. The conversion takes place within the small intestines. For the conversion to be successful, *bile salts and certain enzymes must be present.* Bile salts are only present in the walls of the intestines when one has consumed *fats*. Consequently, **if you have a low-fat diet, it inhibits the body's ability to convert** beta-carotene to vitamin A. A zinc deficiency will also prevent the body from producing the enzymes necessary for the conversion process.

This is the reason that I say one must **consume whole foods and good fats.** It is critical not to consume fractionated foods, because the stomach does not recognize them, and the body receives no nutrition from them. They also wreck digestion. **LOW-fat, NO-fat, anything that takes a food from its natural state and turns it into something unnatural (NOT recognized by the stomach) is not good for the body.**

Back to vitamin A. My heels were nice and smooth when they suddenly developed small cracks on the *outer sides* of the heels. I searched diligently and finally found an article indicating that cracks on the outer side of the heels indicate a vitamin A deficiency, and that one needs to take a vitamin A supplement. The article stated, "25,000 to 50,000 IUs daily"; however, I disagreed. I will tell you why in a moment. I decided to take the minimum that one can find: 10,000 IU tablets. Again, I had to search for a tablet without any other vitamins in it as well as this small IU count. I found Source Naturals Vitamin A (as palmitate) available from both Swanson and Vitacost.

I took one tablet a day after a meal with fats. *Vitamin A is fat soluble.* After about a week, the cracks started to lessen. After a little more than one month, the cracks were disappearing. In another month, they were gone.

Personal Note: Why did I just write "I disagreed"? This is because many years ago I read that vitamin A is very good for the skin and for maintaining a smooth complexion. The general articles advised taking 25,000 IUs daily. I did that. About one year passed, and I suddenly developed flushing skin on my face and chest after ingesting certain fruits, in particular, mangoes, as well as after drinking red wine. The flush would last one to two hours.

I was frantic as I could not figure out what caused this. This was before the Internet. Research meant going to the library and going through medical books, microfilm, and microfiche. Several months elapsed, and I was at home one evening and decided to go through a huge book (in my personal library) called *The Complete Book of Vitamins* (1984) from Rodale Press (which publishes *Prevention* magazine). *THERE IT WAS! An overdose of vitamin A can cause flushing. The body cannot process so much A.*

Do you know how long and hard I had searched for an answer? I also asked a number of doctors, none of whom knew anything. One gave me B12 shots. Another wanted to ply me with creams for my face and chest. One nut wanted to put me on a steroid called prednisone. Ridiculous! The list of side effects is enough to scare one to death. They were so stupid and totally ignorant of body **symptoms**!

I stopped that vitamin A, and the flushing on my chest and cheeks never came back. Therefore, I was leery when reading that I should take a high dose of A for the cracks in my heels. I decided to take the lowest dose available. I took it five days a week and only three weeks a month. It worked, as I wrote, perfectly.

My suggestion to you is to always try a low dose first for any supplement.

DANGER OF LOW-FAT/NO-FAT DIETS
Strokes, Dandruff, Flaking in Eyebrows, Cracks in Skin

Cholesterol IS Important for Our Health

There are numerous references in *Mybyble* to nutrients that are **fat soluble** or **needing fats to convert** them to another nutrient (read previous article "LOW-fat / NO-fat"; beta-carotene **needs fats** in order to convert to vitamin A). Note also that when consuming vegetables (salads) or green drinks, they contain some nutrients that are *fat soluble*. Therefore, one should always have some fat with vegetables (coconut oil is good) in order to digest those nutrients and get nourishment from them.

Are you getting the picture? Many nutrients need fats in the stomach in order to be digested and/or converted into additional vital substances.

The brain, nervous system, and skin certainly need good fats. People on fat-free diets *look* emaciated because they are. Think of former female movie stars and other famous women who were *so* thin and existed on salads. They died too young of diseases, because they failed to provide total nourishment to their bodies which could help prevent disease.

Strokes are connected to deficiencies of fats and vitamin E (which is fat soluble). When the body is deprived of nourishing good fats, it is also devoid of vitamin E and all its components. I use Vitamin Shoppe High Gamma E 400 IU (I have *not* found this exact formulation of E from any other source; one with lunch [you must take it when you are consuming some fats]), Swanson Full Spectrum E with Tocotrienols (one at same time as E), and Selenium L-Selenomethionine 100 mcg (same time as E, from Swanson). These three work synergistically thus providing this nutrient's value. Raw organic nuts and seeds are a fine source of these nutrients but will not provide enough E without supplementation. Aside from **mental lapses** (the brain needs fats to function) perhaps being a symptom of E deficiency, **dandruff in eyebrows or on scalp** is also a **symptom** of a good fats deficiency (and thus E).

Now you surely have the picture. Good fats are needed in order to create additional vital substances and nutrients and keep the body healthy and able to fight off disease.

CHOLESTEROL is not the enemy. Prescription drugs (which drain nutrients) and sugar are the enemies of good health. Cholesterol, a substance required for the normal function of cells, is present in every cell of the human body. It is also found in the bloodstream. This soft, waxy substance is produced in the body and **is essential for the production of vitamin D, bile salts (hence, digestion), and hormones and to protect against infections.** There are scientific articles which propound that **the older a person is, the better a higher cholesterol count is** as opposed to severely low numbers. **The body cannot function optimally with unnatural levels of cholesterol, and that certainly means that the brain and digestion could suffer hugely and traumatically from deficiencies.** Just consider all the obituaries for older people dying from infections. How many of them were on low-cholesterol diets and prescriptions?

There is a general link between low serum cholesterol and increased mortality, particularly in older folks, and there are numerous papers and studies attesting to this.

GOOD FATS, HEALTHY FATS

Mybyble has mentioned sources of good fats which are crucial for good health and names of products that I buy in New York. Goat milk (Oak Knoll), cultured butter (Organic Valley), nonprocessed cheese, organic cage-free eggs (Pete and Gerry's: no pesticides, antibiotics, or GMOs; small family farms; humane treatment), organic coconut oil, organic flax oil, organic beef/game/fowl/pork, safe fish, and numerous other food products provide good fats.

One of the healthiest oils for cooking and baking is Omega Nutrition's **Organic Coconut Oil** which I use on pasta along with their high-lignan **flax oil** and a hefty scoop (included in the canister) of their **Cold-Milled Flax Seeds**. This coconut oil is also perfect for roasting and baking. Grease and baste chickens, turkeys, and potatoes (eaten as an entrée and not improperly combined; see article "Food Combining") for golden, picture-perfect AND HEALTHY finished foods. Sauté onions in this oil by baking them, and then sprinkle on one of **Selina Naturally's** healthful salts. Scramble eggs (having whisked them with goat milk) by placing coconut oil on the pan before scrambling. Enjoy Selina Naturally's **Celtic Sea Salt** on those eggs and her **organic pepper**. I already wrote elsewhere that Omega Nutrition's other coconut oil (virgin) enhances sexual relations, hair and scalp health, should be used for washing the face, and diminished burn freckles on my hand.

Another source would be organic *raw* nuts and seeds. Walnuts, pecans, Brazil nuts, cashews, and **un**pasteurized almonds are wonderful with breakfast or as a snack. They are also delicious when paired with dark chocolate (80 percent cacao and higher are the healthiest chocolates). These nuts are loaded with good fats, vitamins, and minerals. One can go online and look up benefits for each individual nut or seed: sunflower and pumpkin.

Keep this in mind when buying raw organic almonds: you want ***un***pasteurized almonds, including *not* flash pasteurized. Some nuts (pun intended) decided that our healthy US almonds should be pasteurized which results in destroying the nutrient value. I now buy raw organic ***un***pasteurized almonds from two sources: the **Health Nuts** retail store (in a green bag labeled Healthy Nut Factory Organic Raw Almonds Unpasteurized [from Italy]) and also online from **Living Nutz (www.livingnutz.com)**. I also adore shelled raw organic pistachio nuts from both the **Health Nuts** and **Living Nutz**.

Aside from the Health Nuts and Living Nutz, I also buy some raw organic nuts and seeds from Whole Foods. Always make sure that you buy **raw** and **organic**. Roasted and salted will alter the nuts or seeds and impinge upon the nutrient value.

COLDS, COUGHS, SORE THROATS
HAIR DRYER (Great for during Pregnancy), SUPPLEMENTS

Breathe the warm air from a low-watt hair dryer (blower) when you feel that tickle in the throat or slight cough or a sudden runny nose. Long ago, I found that a small, travel-size hair blower is just right for this function.

Sit down and relax (turn on music, television). Angle the blower to get a nice, warm air stream passing the nostrils so that you can breathe in the warm air but not burn your nose. Inhale through the nose for approximately three minutes. Do this every fifteen or twenty minutes, and this will promote a clearing of the nasal passage very quickly.

The warm air from the dryer is heated to just the point that it kills germs in the mucous membranes and opens nasal passages. Repeat treatments reinforce each other, and relief will follow. One can even carry this small travel blower to the office.

This treatment is also so useful to someone who is **PREGNANT** and not taking medication. Catch a cold, cough, or sore throat early—at its incipient moment—and often one can short-circuit it with this nontoxic solution.

If I feel sniffles or a tickle in my throat, I sit in my bathroom where I have my small hair blower, turn on my radio, and give myself several minutes' treatment.

SUPPLEMENTS: The *moment* that one feels that tickle or sniffle, **that** is the time to act! Take Standard Process **Congaplex** (three capsules the first dose; then each hour for up to five hours, two capsules per hour). **Echinacea (HERE IS VITAL INFORMATION):** So many people whine that Echinacea does not work. That is because **it must be taken *correctly* in order to get tissue saturation.** One **must take three capsules every two hours for *just* six hours**. That means **that in six hours, one will have taken one's total allotment of nine capsules** for the day. This will give the respiratory system the support that it needs **along with the other supplements** in this protocol. **Pau d'Arco**: Take exactly as Echinacea and at the same time. **Kyolic Garlic Formula 100** capsules: Take two caps three times daily with meals. Kyolic Garlic is both a huge preventive as well as therapeutic boost. I use it almost every day (five days a week and three weeks per month; I give myself some days off "for good behavior"; actually, to allow the body to clear out and start fresh). Kyolic has been used in many studies of the benefits of garlic. It does *not* give you garlic breath. Importantly, **garlic is a natural detoxifier,** including for lead poisoning. It is not only as effective as a common chelation drug in pulling lead out of the body but also much safer.

NutriBiotic Grapefruit Seed Extract (GSE): Written about in several *Mybyble* articles, GSE is almost thirty years old. As an antimicrobial, antibacterial, antiviral, and antifungal product, I use fifteen drops which is the therapeutic dose (stirred into pure water), three times daily. I use it to take some of these supplements. A preventive dose is five drops three times daily. You might ask, What does it taste like? Answer: The new formula has almost no taste. Perhaps it tastes like a drop of grapefruit squeezed into water. This also functions as a gargle. I keep a two-ounce bottle with me at all times and never fly without using it. It also is good for protection if one must visit someone in a hospital.

Honey and apple cider vinegar (see *Mybyble* article and follow directions) is a must! Drink it all day long. One can also gargle with this soothing drink.

Twice in twenty-eight years I became infected with a horrendous cough. It came from deep in the chest and caused immense mucus to be produced and expectorated. Once was from being in an airplane and then a restaurant suffused with cigarette smoke and coughing people. That was twenty-eight years back. I felt that I had walking pneumonia. The second time was in December 2012. On Christmas Eve we sat in front of some people (at a midnight Christmas Carol service) who hacked away. I turned and asked them, "How sick are you?" They were tourists from Southeast Asia and said that they had "picked up some violent cough". By the next evening, I was infected badly. In such a situation, I **add two supplements** to the protocol just listed: **Olive Leaf Extract** (500 mg) and **Prickly Pear Cactus** Opuntia (650 mg), and I even took three additional **Echinacea** in the evening (hours after the original nine capsules). I used a tablespoon of **raw honey** with a teaspoon of **apple cider vinegar** in a mug of warm pure water every hour for six hours, because it eased the coughing and helped heal my respiratory system while the supplements did their work. Tissue saturation with the supplements is critical in such a situation.

There is an **excellent lozenge** to use for dry, tickly, sore, or strained throats. **Thayers Slippery Elm Lozenges** come in natural (my preference) as well as flavors. Take them with you to the movies, theater, business meetings, on airplanes. Always keep a couple handy. It is an immediately soothing remedy that has been available since 1847! It soothes mouth and throat tissues *without* menthol.

One can also **gargle** with Celtic Sea Salt. Any of the natural gargles mentioned in this article can be used all day long in order to help the throat win the battle against soreness.

Do not be overwhelmed. Reread the article. Making notes and a list is helpful, because writing this down puts it more permanently in your head. Reread the article several days from now. These supplements should always be in one's home for immediate use.

VETERINARIAN PRODUCTS, ANIMALS

There are numerous mentions of Standard Process products in *Mybyble*. Please note that they also have a significant veterinarian product line as well as children's products. These supplements are with whole-food ingredients which support the body. Animals know whole food. They suffer terribly (just as humans do) when eating processed food which provides no nourishment.

Personal Note: Beau (our standard poodle as I grew up) loved when Grandma (a brilliant chef) would be making chicken soup and roast chicken. He could smell (of course) what was cooking, and he would sit for several hours in the kitchen at Grandma's feet while she cleaned the chicken and prepared the giblets. Beau knew that he was getting all the giblets. Grandma cooked everything to perfection, and when all was removed from the stove and oven, she would place what Beau was getting into his dinner bowl and leave it on the counter to cool. She would pat Beau and say, "OK, Beau. Just a few minutes and it will be ready for you." Beau would just sit there and wait. Then he would lap up that scrumptious whole food. I now understand much better than I did then what it means for a doggy to have fresh food. Their digestion, coat, and immune system function wonderfully on real food.

I assure you that totally **whole-food supplements work for people and for pets**. Take an enjoyable and informative look at the easy-to-navigate Standard Process site. See "Source List".

CLEARING SINUSES
The Ultimate Solution

Breathing Bad Air, Rash on Face or Body, Beginning of a Cold

I was twenty-two years old and working for the fifth largest medical center in the metropolitan New York area. I was walking down one of our hospital's hallways (we had three hospitals) and suffering from an awful sinus headache. Hence, I had my hand to the side of my head because it was throbbing so badly.

A doctor passed and suddenly called to me, saying, "Hello. Excuse me." I turned to him, and he smiled, saying, "You are having a sinus headache?" I said that it was just awful and that I had them a couple of times a month. He said, "Come with me. My office is just down the hall." We went in, and he started explaining what he would prescribe for me. I immediately interrupted and said that I had no interest in little tablets or nose sprays, because they were useless and only created a rebound effect.

He looked right at me and said, "Do I look like a quack? I do not prescribe such nonsense. I am chief of allergies and immunology, and I agree with you, those other things are *not* a cure. What I am giving you is a lifetime solution to what causes the headache . . . which is **clogged sinuses**." I just loved hearing "Do I look like a quack?" That is exactly what I considered anyone who prescribed those **over-the-counter tablets and nose sprays. They do not cure, but they create a** rebound effect which means that the stuffiness and sniffles come back worse than before.

The doctor wrote a prescription for *salt water!* In actual fact, it was for **normal saline solution 0.9% Sodium Chloride Irrigation** USP in a 500 mL bottle. He told me that the pharmacy would also give me a small bottle with a *three-inch eyedropper*. I could transfer the saline solution into that bottle. This is still a prescription item in New York.

The **simple cleansing procedure** is as follows: Transfer saline into the smaller bottle, fill the eyedropper, and (standing at your bathroom sink) flush your nostrils (head tilted back). Use three droppers-full per nostril, each one pointing in a different direction and thus toward different sinuses—point up, down, and sideways. You need to reach ALL the sinuses. Expectorate (spit out what trickles down into the throat). Blow the nose 'real good'. **Do this twice to three times per day for one or two weeks, and that should do it. You may never have sinus trouble again.**

One can enhance the effectiveness of saline solution by using Echinacea, Kyolic Garlic, and NutriBiotic Grapefruit Seed Extract. See article "Colds, Coughs, Sore Throats".

For years, I carried saline solution when I travelled; however, I never needed it for a sinus headache again.

I do use saline solution from time to time, though, when I come home from Manhattan after a particularly dusty day or if I breathed in some bad air near a construction site. I was at my Wall Street office when the United States was attacked on September 11, 2001. I was there for two days. Once I finally got home, I certainly used saline solution once a day for several days in order to cleanse my sinuses and get rid of bacteria.

When I developed a **rash** on my face from some bacteria, I flushed my nose with saline in order to help the healing process. I recommended this to someone with **rosacea**, and he said that he noticed a definite reduction in redness and breakouts.

HOW TO GARGLE (especially for SORE THROATS)

In order to be effective, any **gargle must be held in the throat for thirty seconds**. Gargle gently. If you cannot hold it for thirty seconds, tilt the head forward while keeping the liquid in your mouth, get a breath through your nose, then tilt the head back, and continue to gargle. The **sore or infected throat must have sustained contact with the germ killer.**

GARGLES
Sore Throat, Overused Voice

There are several gargles that are useful when something attacks the throat. Depending upon what is causing the troubled throat, one or another of these gargles could be a solution. Of course, **for an overused voice, one needs soothing number 4 or 5**.

1. Nutribiotic Grapefruit Seed Extract. In two fingers or less of warm or room temperature pure water, place four to five drops. Stir in order to disperse the drops. Gargle (see instructions in "Gargle—Sore Throats" article). This product can also be drunk, so it is fine if some is swallowed.
2. Amber (my preference) or blue or green disinfectant gargle. The house brand of any drugstore is fine. I buy this from CVS, and it is called CVS Antiseptic Gargle. Use it full strength. Follow instructions in "Gargle—Sore Throats". I find this an excellent remedy, especially at the incipient tickle or scratchiness.
3. Hydrogen peroxide 3%. One-half teaspoon in two fingers warm or room temperature pure water. Peroxide naturally fizzes, so be prepared for the fizz.
4. George's Always Active® Aloe Vera (I purchase it by the gallon and put small amounts in little bottles, such as empty vitamin bottles or small water bottles). Use it full strength. **This is also very soothing for an overused voice. Gargle gently.** Since this product is drinkable, one can either swallow what is gargled or not worry if some trickles down the throat. It tastes just like spring water.

5. Honey and apple cider vinegar. See following article, "Honey and Apple Cider Vinegar", for details. One can gargle with just <u>raw</u> organic honey in warm pure water (one tablespoon per mug of warm water; this will last for many hours of gargling), or one can add *less* than a teaspoon of organic, raw, unfiltered apple cider vinegar to the mug in order to get those healing properties of both ingredients working together.
6. Celtic Sea Salt. Stir a teaspoon of (Selina Naturally) chunky light grey into a mug of pure water and stir. It can be kept handy all day in order to take a small mouthful and gargle.

Try each of these remedies to see which suits the malady of the moment. All these items should always be in the home.

HONEY AND APPLE CIDER VINEGAR
Coughs, Colds, Bladder Problems, Kidney Problems, Urination Problems

When using honey, it is the **organic <u>raw</u>** honey that provides the maximum nutrients. It is a joy when one can buy local honey that is raw and organic; however, since that is not available where I live, I buy Y.S. Organic Bee Farms Raw Honey.

Never refrigerate honey or apple cider vinegar. They are stable at room temperature. Raw honey changes its consistency depending upon temperature. I keep the jar that I am using near my stove, as the warmth will keep the honey easy to spoon out. **Should you suddenly need honey from a jar where the product is solid, take your metal tablespoon, run it under very hot water** (better still, boil a cup of water and stand the spoon in that water for several seconds), dry the spoon, and **that nice, hot spoon will slide into the solid honey perfectly.**

The most nutritious honeys are the darker honeys. Buckwheat and alfalfa are particularly good as well as being amongst the most nutritious. Darker buckwheat has the most minerals while alfalfa has roots that go deeper into the ground than any other, thereby giving a nutrient-rich product. The two honeys also combine nicely in a mug of water.

Per mug of warm pure water, add one full tablespoon of honey plus one teaspoon of apple cider vinegar (ACV), or to your taste. You can make several cups in advance and cover the top of the cup with an old plastic cover or similar. This is a useful procedure when you are using the honey to both drink and gargle. It saves time by not needing to make each cup over and over.

Honey and ACV are antibacterial and antimicrobial, and therefore the drink will not spoil even if sitting on the counter for a couple of days. Microwave it for twenty to thirty seconds (depending upon one's microwave) to warm it or, better still (I prefer this method as it does not alter the enzymes), heat it in a small pot on the stove. Hold the pot *above* the flame (*not* on it) as you only want to warm it.

At the first hint of a cough, or certainly once a cough has fully blossomed, drink this every hour (or every ninety minutes) in order to saturate the lungs and respiratory system with nutrients flowing through the body. Do this five times. With a serious infection, one needs to do this every forty-five minutes five times. If you are away from home, any honey with fresh lemon will suffice temporarily. Should you be staying in a hotel, the chef for the dining room almost always has a supply of honey. Get some (as well as lemon) to keep in your room.

Personal Note: When I first started **taking herbs, I overdid it!** That caused me to **urinate too frequently** due to overuse of herbal capsules over a long period of time which **put pressure on my bladder and kidneys**. I stopped taking the herbs but still sought a natural healing solution. Good fortune smiled upon me as the Museum of Natural History in Manhattan was having a guest lecturer one Sunday morning. He was a doctor from Singapore, and he specialized in natural medicine. I immediately responded to the invitation. Everyone in the audience (of about sixty people) was given a number, and if your number was chosen, you would be one of the handful of attendees to have a private reading from the doctor. I was one of those lucky people; I was also the last one chosen.

I sat across from the doctor. He had me remove my jewelry and put my elbows on the table and stretch my arms across to him. He held my hands, ran his fingertips up and down my arms (to feel how my blood was running, he told me), felt my pulse, and also felt my neck. He then told me that I took too many herbs (for too long), that my "blood was racing", and that I needed to tone my bladder and kidneys. He wrote down—in Chinese—several items for me to purchase in Chinatown (downtown in Manhattan), as well as to **use honey, bee propolis, and alfalfa**. This man was sent to me—at that moment—from heaven. That was just how I felt.

I thoroughly investigated what I should use for **toning those organs**. They had been stressed due to my lengthy overuse of herbs which I had been taking because of menstrual cramps.

Honey, ACV, bee propolis, and alfalfa (both tablets and honey) tone internal organs and are especially beneficial to the kidneys and bladder, the doctor explained to me. I used a mug of honey and ACV upon arising and before going to bed, as well as spacing out during the day the following: alfalfa tablets (10 grain [650 mg] tablets from Puritan's Pride), taking two tablets three times daily; bee propolis (from Swanson or Puritan's Pride), taking 1,000 mg three times daily; and drinking six ounces daily of George's Always Active® Aloe Vera (purchased from the Health Nuts and also from Vitacost).

Over a number of months, the honey, ACV, alfalfa, and bee propolis completely stopped the **urination problem: no arising at night and no running to bathrooms all day. It was quite a lesson.**

NODULES ON VOCAL CORDS
Strained Voice, Overused Voice

A singer once told me that he had some nodules on his vocal cords. A doctor wanted to operate; however, this man sought a natural solution as he was not enthusiastic about having anyone cut around his vocal cords.

He consulted a voice coach and was told to sip honey (in a mug of water) all day long, to let it slowly go down the throat, to not eat anything when doing this, and to just let the honey water (see *Mybyble* article "Honey and Apple Cider Vinegar") saturate the throat without interference from other food or drink.

He diligently did this and also used his voice as little as possible. After a number of months, the nodules were gone. Remember, too, that **when the voice is stressed, you do *not* want to speak in a lower pitch than your normal pitch because *that* stresses the voice even more**. Just refrain from unnecessary talk. Let the voice rest, keep hydrated with pure water, and sip honey water, which tones and heals. (See article "Hum for Healthy Vocal Cords")

TEETH, GUMS, DENTISTS

When you have any dental work done, take a small bottle of **George's Always Active® Aloe Vera** with you so that you can swoosh with it before leaving the dentist's office. It is soothing and healing. Keep it in your mouth for a few minutes before expectorating.

Keep aloe in your office or home in order to swoosh during the day. Swoosh on airplanes after a long flight. Certainly **drink it for enhanced digestion.**

COLLAGEN OR JUVÉDERM INJECTIONS

When going for facial injections for wrinkles, bring a small bottle of **George's Always Active® Aloe Vera**. Put some on a gauze pad, and pat it onto the entry sites just after the doctor injects you. It is far kinder to the skin than alcohol and also promotes healing/closure of the injection marks.

Taking a tablet of **bromelain** just before the injections is also supportive. Bromelain reduces inflammation and bleeding. Note that bromelain acts as an anti-inflammatory when taken *between* meals; however, if taken *with* a meal, it acts as a digestive. The reason is because bromelain goes to the site of activity in the body. If one is eating, then digestion is the activity, and bromelain will focus on that.

If there is an injury and bleeding, bromelain will go there and act to stop bleeding and reduce inflammation.

After the injections, stir five drops of **NutriBiotic Grapefruit Seed Extract** into a small cup of pure water. Dab it all over the injection site in order to clean up any bacteria. Then drink the treated water. No matter how careful a doctor is, bacteria could still be present and can cause itching. The grapefruit seed extract is a wonderful preventive.

For several days before the injections, one should *not* take any capsules or tablets that thin the blood, because that will cause more bleeding and bruising. Garlic, vitamin E, certain herbs, and fish oil should be avoided for three days prior to the procedure; however, taking **vitamin K2** (see "Source List" for what I buy; see *Mybyble* article "Heart Palpitations and Arrhythmias" for full information on K2) **can be very helpful in preventing bleeding**. **Horsetail** capsules are also coagulants and can help prevent bruising and bleeding. Horsetail can be taken for three days before injections with the final capsule on the day of the injections.

"DON'T PICK!"—and Other Bon Mots from Mom

As my mother always said—and the older I get, the more she is proven right—"Don't pick at pimples or anything!", "Don't squeeze", "Don't frown", "Don't squint".

Let me tell you, the first wrinkles you will see are where you squeezed pimples. Frown marks will suddenly appear if you are a frowner. If you had sunburn, that is where you will have freckles and moles. On the face, collagen is destroyed by *over*sunning. **Sun itself is good for the body**. One just must not burn.

Frown—and other facial mismanagement—prevention: Just watch other people's faces. You will see their frowning, raising of eyebrows and wrinkling the forehead, excessively moving the lips, and creating wrinkles. **Other people's faces are a mirror for your viewing, and *they* act as preventives** for your not forming those habits **OR** to remind you *not* to do that!

HORSERADISH
STOMACH, LIVER, GENERAL HEALTH

Enjoy a nice half teaspoon (or more) of **horseradish** every day. It is good for the **stomach, liver, heart,** and more and is a **cancer fighter**. I buy Gold's red horseradish because that is the taste that I enjoy. Additionally, a few years back, I had a question about horseradish, and I called Gold's headquarters in Hempstead, New York (on Long Island). What a pleasure to find **an American company** founded in 1932 by the grandparents of the current owners, and one of the principals of the company got on the telephone to speak with me. They take pride in the same recipe from inception. The Journal of Agricultural and Food Chemistry found that horseradish contains <u>ten times *more*</u> detoxifying chemicals than broccoli, which slow the growth of tumors and help the liver eliminate carcinogens. Even one-quarter teaspoon per day is beneficial.

The use of this herb goes back in history. There are numerous preventive and therapeutic uses for digestion, teeth and gums, respiratory system (clearing mucus), pain, and more. It has no fat, no cholesterol, almost no calories, is low in sodium, and contains vitamins, minerals, and antioxidants. Enjoy a small amount before, during, or after any meal.

Also note that <u>*freshly grated horseradish*</u> is a joy. There is a favorite restaurant of mine which grates fresh horseradish for my oysters. At home, I do not have the time, and I use Gold's.

Personal Note: I found this horseradish to be healing for my stomach after I was poisoned by a defective pot. See article "Are Pots and Pans Poisoning You?"

HANGOVER? A LITTLE TOO MUCH ALCOHOL? STOMACH SICK? POISONING from Food or Other? OVERDOSE?

There are three remedies for overdone drinking—whether way too much or just a bit. The first is to **drink a lot of pure water**. I write *pure* because it should **not** contain fluoride or chlorine. You need water free of toxic contaminants when treating overdrinking so that the water gets right into your system and is not stymied by inorganic material. If one consumes eight ounces of water for every ounce of liquor, it will help flush the system. If water was not consumed while drinking, drink a lot later.

Secondly, take one or two **charcoal capsules**. One capsule will open in the stomach to massive size. It sops up **poisons—and most everything**—in the stomach (including some of the liquor that has not yet been introduced into the bloodstream), as well as fats. **One should never drink without having fatty foods in the stomach,** because they slow the body's absorption of alcohol! Then if one takes charcoal, it can sop up those fatty foods, which will also contain some of that alcohol.

In the case of poison, activated charcoal attaches to the poison and prevents its absorption in the stomach. It is critical, though, to know with which **poison (drugs, liquor, or other**) you are dealing in order to effect correct treatment. Call Poison Control for help. Always have activated charcoal capsules in your home. I buy them from Puritan's Pride (#3680). They have a good shelf life, but since a poisoning emergency is almost nonexistent, I discard the expired and buy new ones. Note that if one uses charcoal frequently, you will need to take vitamin/mineral supplements in order to replace what gets eliminated, as vitamins and nutrients in the stomach will be sopped up by the charcoal.

Thirdly, after too much drinking, there is **honey and apple cider vinegar**. See the *Mybyble* article. You will need at least one mug, if not more. It truly helps.

ARE POTS AND PANS POISONING YOU?
Nausea, Chest Pain/Constriction, Inexplicable Rash, Eyebrows Curling

If you have intermittent nausea during the day and sometimes get chest discomfort (and even tight constriction which passes after a few minutes), check the pots with which you are cooking and also boiling water for tea or coffee. In particular, check those sealed tea kettles that whistle and pots with no-stick film. You may be getting poisoned.

Pots that have those no-stick film interiors can start to deteriorate over the years, and infinitesimal flakes get into boiling water or food. As you ingest that, you are ingesting poison which accumulates in your system. There are subtle warnings: an inexplicable hive (for example, on the lower spine near the buttocks) or rash, definitely any rash on the face where the pores seem to erupt (including by the eyebrows and hairline) similar to rosacea, bumps under the skin, nauseousness after eating or drinking something from those pots. Do **NOT** use pots with scratches, nicks, or no-stick film. Do NOT use sealed pots (like whistling kettles) where you cannot view the interior.

Personal Note: When I first worked in a major medical center after I graduated from New York University, my office was right down the hall from a little kitchen. There was a **whistling tea kettle** which we all used to boil water. I would go to work feeling fine; however, **by late afternoon, my stomach would be deathly sick**. Driving home, I always felt that I would throw up. After I had dinner, the upset would subside until the next day. Some time went by, and then in my office, I suffered **horrendous chest constrictions**. I thought that I was having a heart attack. I was twenty-one years old. I rested my head on my desk for about twenty minutes, and then it passed. Also, my **eyebrows started to curl** at the ends just a tiny bit. One afternoon, I heard a big crash and walked out to the kitchen where someone was gasping. She had dropped the tea kettle, and the whole whistling top broke off, and the kettle split in half. Horror of all horrors, **the inside was totally corroded and filled with rust! We were slowly being poisoned.** Within two weeks, my eyebrows started to grow correctly, my stomach was back to normal, and that face rash (I had thought that I was suddenly getting acne) disappeared.

Fast forward twenty-five years, and suddenly I developed a face rash, bumps, chest pains, and nauseousness. It went on for weeks as I kept eliminating possible offending items. Suddenly I remembered the rusting tea pot, and I thought, *I am boiling water for my tea in a glass pot with a black no-stick film interior, and I had noticed that that film started looking as though it was flaking off.* All the horror of viewing that corroded tea kettle came back to me. I threw out the glass pot and called Poison Control. It took several calls to find a woman with knowledge of poisoning via no-stick glass pots, but I found one. She said that I definitely was affected by that pot and that I should drink two gallons of pure water a day in order to flush my system, take charcoal but only for a few days (because it also swallows up nutrients that are in one's stomach), and take garlic.

See previous article "Hangover . . . Poisoning". Once I realized that I was being poisoned—both currently and twenty-five years earlier—I used **charcoal** capsules and all the remedies in this article to support my body's recuperation. **Horseradish** (see article) also helped my stomach. **Kyolic Garlic** was **very, very** helpful as well. It is a natural detoxifier. See "Colds, Coughs, Sore Throats" article.

DANDRUFF, DRY HAIR AFTER SHAMPOO

In order to restore pH balance after one shampoos, use Omega Nutrition's Organic Unfiltered Apple Cider Vinegar. Prepare in a nonbreakable bottle one-third cup ACV to one quart water. You can also use a smaller bottle for water and proportionately reduce the ACV. Keep it in your bathroom. After you wash out the shampoo, shake the ACV bottle and gently dribble it all over the scalp. Then proceed to dry as usual. You will find hair easier to comb and dry, and the **scalp and follicles** will benefit from this nourishing treatment. This ACV protocol along with Wholemega Fish Oil (see *Mybyble* article) is an excellent treatment for **dandruff.**

CHILL IT! ICING WINE

If you need to quickly chill champagne, white wine, beer, or any drink, **add salt to the ice** bucket. Put the bottle into a bucket of ice *and* water, then spread a cup of table salt all over the top of the ice around the bottle, and push some salt down into the ice water by the bottle. It will chill within twelve to fifteen minutes depending upon the size of the bottle. If it is a very small bottle, it may be chilled more quickly. A toast to your health!

MYBYBLE

RECORKING AN OPEN BOTTLE OF WINE

Years back, in Europe, a wonderful chef taught me the trick of perfectly and easily corking an opened bottle of wine. It even works with champagne. You need to have on hand a selection of corks from former bottles, and the *best ones* are from sherry bottles or champagne because they have the little affixed tops, which make them sturdier and easier to grip. Ask the bartender at your favorite restaurant to save a bunch of corks for you. He/she will be delighted.

Once you open a wine, select a cork that will go into the top air-tight, because you are going to **turn the bottle upside down,** and one does not want any leaking. Sometimes one can use the wine's own cork by reversing it and putting the topside in first. Rarely, though, does that work because the cork may have cracked when being opened.

Once you have the right cork size, test for leaks by laying the bottle in your kitchen sink or standing it upside down in a pot. Once you know it is safe, select a nice, quiet corner on your countertop, place a mug or small container there, and stand the bottle upside down in it, resting it against the wall. You get the idea. Find a spot where the bottle can balance against something in order to be kept upright and not slide or fall.

My wines can last two to three weeks this way, as I drink just a minor amount with dinner. Since I drink nice wines, I want to enjoy to the last drop.

For white wines or champagne, find the right spot in the refrigerator to lay the bottle down, and keep the cork wet. Preferably, use a vegetable <u>drawer</u> just in case it leaks.

SLEEP PROBLEMS, INSOMNIA, RESTLESS LEGS

Falling asleep, staying asleep, or falling back to sleep if awakened (to urinate, for example) are significant troubles for many. There are different solutions/remedies that work at varying times. I will offer <u>every</u> aid that has worked for me. Once upon a time, I slept like a log—solid! As time went on, business and personal stress as well as nutrient deficiencies sometimes interfered with my sleep patterns. Here are solutions:

> First, get **morning sunlight** shining onto your face. Do not look straight at the sun, but try to step out on a terrace or open a window (you cannot stand *behind* the window because it blocks the rays, which must hit the body) so that you can get ten minutes (or more) of sun, which helps to set your body clock. This goes back to our origins when people arose at sunrise and went to sleep at sunset. Use these minutes to do arm isometrics or cross-crawl standing in place (see the *Mybyble* articles).

> Secondly, be sure that you have *no* lights in the bedroom. Cover any digital clock or air-conditioner temperature monitor with a cloth. The room must be dark. Keep a **flashlight** by the bed in case you wake to urinate. You do not want to turn on a bright light and disturb your mental state. Move the clock radio away from the head of the bed. Also, **do not use electric blankets**. These too affect the body *extremely* adversely just as computers or power wires do, which bombard us with electromagnetic waves all day long. **No computers** before bedtime. Just because you cannot *see* these dangerous waves does not mean that they are not there and doing terrible harm to the body.

> Thirdly, **breathe**. Lie on your back. Close your eyes. Breathe in slowly as though "blowing up a balloon" in your tummy. Hold your breath. Release through the mouth. Do this twenty times and *focus* on the breathing. Do not think of other things.

> Fourthly, there are four **supplements** that I have found very useful:
> 1. Standard Process **Min-Tran**: Many people are deficient in minerals that are critical to calming the

body. Min-Tran is a vegetarian product that contains mineral complexes to support emotional balance. It is a mild calmative that helps ease stress. One should take six tablets three times daily with the final six right at bedtime (and the middle six around four hours prior to bedtime). See if that works over a month's time. If this is successful, you can reduce the number to five (three times daily) and then four. You can also see if four at dinnertime and five at bedtime do the trick. (You will also note improved fingernails as these minerals enhance nails.)

2. Standard Process **Cruciferous Complete**: Some sleep issues are due to hormone imbalances. Excess estrogen in women can cause sleep problems. Cruciferous vegetables are a wonderful remedy. This product is food based from kale and brussels sprouts and is a source of vitamin K, which supports calcium absorption, blood clotting, and healthy liver function. It contains trace amounts of lutein, which, in higher amounts, appears to support healthy eye function. Take one capsule before dinner. Along with Min-Tran, this duo can help.

3. **Suntheanine L-Theanine** (bought from Swanson): This product is a unique amino acid derived from green tea leaves, which reduces nervous tension and promotes relaxation. One 100 mg capsule before bedtime can promote sleep. I have found it useful many times but not always.

4. **L-Tryptophan TryptoPure** (from Swanson) is stronger and is a precursor to serotonin, which helps us fall asleep and stay asleep. It is an essential amino acid and supports against nervousness and tension. I find this the most reliable for giving me a full night's sleep. Take one capsule thirty to sixty minutes before sleeping. Two capsules will provide stronger benefit. Try one the first time. If that is successful, one does not need two.

When I feel that my sleeping will need help, I use one L-Tryptophan. This is *not* every night; however, Min-Tran and Cruciferous Complete are healthful food supplements that also promote good sleep. I use them almost every day.

RESTLESS LEGS: This debilitating, sleep-invading aggravation is caused by a nutrient deficiency. Which nutrients depend upon the person and what his/her body is lacking. It is, though, one of two nutrient groups. Both are discussed in "Palpitations . . . Cough to Get You Heart Beating" article. It is either a lack in calcium, magnesium, D3, K or a lack in the B vitamins group or both.

VENOUS INSUFFICIENCY, CIRCULATION, HEMORRHOIDS
Tone Inner Thighs and Buttocks (see end of article)

A wonderful doctor diagnosed my mild venous insufficiency in my left leg and told me that a new surgical procedure—done in his office—would fix it. He said, "Carole, I know you believe in vitamins and herbs, but this is one condition that you cannot treat that way." I would not consider the surgery as I have never been under anesthesia and did not want to subject my body to that now.

I went home and immediately started to research "venous insufficiency". This took weeks. I matched appropriate supplements to the problem and started treatment, and then it took months of refining what I tried. I finally had the products listed below, which addressed my condition and worked synergistically to remedy it. Within a couple of days, I no longer had **tired legs** or **redness on the top** of my left foot after a full day at business. Gone was the **puffiness** on top of that left foot as well, nor did I have discomfort anymore when sleeping.

It is now ten years since the diagnosis. See the "Source List" for product information. Here is what I use (in conjunction with my daily supplement protocol):

1. Standard Process **Vasculin** (#8165). Strong on **niacin (which thins the blood and promotes eased circulation)** plus B vitamins and other nutrients. Whole food-based. I always take two at bedtime, which relaxes my left leg perfectly. I

also take them during a long business day in order to keep my circulation perfect.

2. Standard Process **Circuplex** (#2650). Promotes healthy peripheral circulation and vascular integrity. One capsule has much more niacin than one Vasculin. At the beginning, I needed this stronger capsule desperately. Once I integrated all the products that I list here, I no longer needed Circuplex. I always believe in using as few products as possible and at the lowest dose possible which accomplishes the task.

3. I also use Standard Process **Cataplex B** (#1250) and **Cardio-Plus** (#2080) for a total B protocol as well as the tablets' additional niacin. View complete information on website (see "Source List").

4. **DiosVein** (SWU720 from Swanson) combines diosmin and hesperidin. Diosmin improves blood **circulation** and **strengthens vein walls** by improving the **elasticity** of blood vessels while inhibiting certain proinflammatory lipids. Diosmin **helps blood** to **flow against gravity and return from the legs to the heart**. This has the effect of **reducing varicose and spider veins** while preventing recurrence by treating their cause. Diosmin has been shown to relieve painful **hemorrhoid symptoms,** which can be caused by an enlarged varicose vein in the rectal area. For my venous insufficiency, DiosVein was an invaluable find in my "Health Sciences Institute" newsletter. (See article "Learn"). **Dose** *schedule*: Initially, I took three per day five days a week. Once I was having relief with my left leg, I went to two capsules daily. This works perfectly. I give myself off two days a week as well as the first week of every month. Additionally, after two months, I stop taking DiosVein for four to six weeks. I read this suggestion in an article and could understand that it is beneficial to clear certain products from the body. Then when one restarts them, they have the fresh power to heal.

Hesperidin is in DiosVein and is a derivative of citrus fruits, mainly vitamin C found in oranges. Allergic reactions and malabsorption are possible in sensitive individuals, such as itching, hives, and a rash. Individuals who have been diagnosed as intolerant or allergic to fructose should avoid using hesperidin.

5. For those with **hemorrhoids or rectal irritation**, it is also easing and healing to gently **insert emu oil into the rectum**. Wear a thin rubber surgical glove, put emu all over a fingertip, and introduce it into the affected area. One may need to do this two or three times in order to coat the internal area. Repeat all day as needed.

6. **Horse Chestnut** (#NSI 3005796 from Vitacost). I take one capsule two times daily with the same days off as described in DiosVein. It can be taken in small doses and is a traditional remedy for leg vein health. It tones and protects blood vessels and may be helpful in ankle edema (swelling) related to poor venous return. Horse chestnut is an astringent, anti-inflammatory herb that helps to tone the vein walls, which, when slack or distended, may become varicose, hemorrhoidal, or otherwise problematic. The plant also reduces fluid retention by increasing the permeability of the capillaries and allowing the reabsorption of excess fluid back into the circulatory system.

7. **Swanson Grapeseed, Green Tea & Pine Bark Complex** (SW1024). Each capsule contains a significant 125 mg of each ingredient. It is unusual to find this complex, which I discovered when seeking a product less costly than pycnogenol (derived from pine bark). I take one capsule twice daily (one around noon and one late afternoon) and have found it to integrate nicely with my other supplements. Same *schedule* as written before.

8. **Puritan's Pride Grape Extract** 60 mg (#6317) from skin *and* seed plus resveratrol and ellagic acid. There is strong evidence that grape seed extract is beneficial for a number of cardiovascular conditions and may help with a type of poor circulation (chronic venous insufficiency) and high cholesterol.

This grape is the muscadine grape (*Vitis rotundifolia*), which has numerous health benefits and helps blood health, reducing oxidative stress to the heart by helping to reduce inflammation to blood vessels, thus reducing atherosclerotic plaque formation. I take one capsule with dinner per the schedule to which I previously referred.

9. **Compression hose**. The doctor who diagnosed my condition did make a superb suggestion: use compression hose. He suggested Sigvaris, and I prefer the style that is closed toe and comes up to the midthigh. There are also open toe and knee-high. I buy them from three discount companies: www.compressionsale.com, www.discountsurgical.com, and www.foryourlegs.com. They each have various sales as well as new-customer discounts if one signs up online to receive e-mails. When you telephone, the staff is very knowledgeable and helpful. It is very important to **remember the following**: *First*, **wear rubber gloves** when putting on the hose. Otherwise, you abrade the pads of your fingers and could also catch your fingernails. I use thin surgical gloves about which I previously wrote in *Mybyble*. *Secondly*, **lie on your bed**, put legs up, and pull on hose from that position and **not** from a standing position, **because** you want to have the blood flowing toward the heart and not pooled down around the ankles. THIS IS AN INCREDIBLE TIP. No one tells you this. It is also easier to get them on from a reclining position. *Thirdly*, I like to have **two strengths** to choose between when I come home from business and pull on the hose just for comfort. When you read the sites for these hose, you will note that there is 20-30 mmHg for *medium support* and 15-20 mmHg for *mild (or light) support*. Sometimes, I want the light support, so I have the Sigvaris EverSheer 781N. For a heavier hose (more like tights), I use Sigvaris 862N in the medium support.

The 862N also has more durability than the EverSheer. These are available **for both women and men.** My venous insufficiency is under such good control that I can easily also just use **regular pantyhose**. I buy "East 5th Sheer Caress

Sheerest Support" from JCPenney. They have a beautiful, silky sheen and are stunning hose (in a number of shades)!

IMPORTANT CIRCULATION TIP: When one is not wearing compression hose or pantyhose and the legs are getting heavy or twitchy, here is something to help whether one is sitting or standing: Squeeze the legs from the ankles up through the thighs and buttocks. <u>*Tighten*</u> *all the muscles. The aim is to get circulation moving the blood from the ankles back to the heart.* Therefore, tightening, holding, releasing, and tightening again helps to do that. I find it of great value. When you are sitting and doing this tightening, you can **add the benefit of isometrics**. Put your ankles together but the knees splayed (outward). Then tighten the thighs and buttocks while *pretending* to bring the knees together. You do *not* want to close the knees. You only want to create the healing **tension**. This stimulates the circulation. It is also **excellent for toning the inner thighs especially and the buttocks. One can do this isometric anywhere.**

TRAVELLING

Travels, both for business and pleasure, can be stressful. **A good multinutrient** can boost the immune system. I use Standard Process Immuplex (two caps three times daily) when travelling. I also use Immuplex—if there is a sudden tickle, sniffle, or cough—along with Congaplex. (See "Coughs, Colds" article.)

TRAVEL: HOTEL ROOMS, BATHROOMS

Travelling is more risky today. Germs pervade most areas we inhabit, and taking precautions is the wisest move in order to prevent illness when travelling.

The hotel room is a key spot on which to focus. **CRITICAL:** Wash (do this yourself) any glasses from which you drink! *Use normal soap* (**not** antibacterial; see *Mybyble* article "Washing Fruits and Vegetables: Never Antibacterial"), and give glasses a good washing. If you are staying longer than one day, tell housekeeping **not** to touch your glasses! **WHY?** In more than one deluxe hotel in the world, I have found maids putting glasses in the bathroom sink and rinsing them with the same dirty gloved hands used to clean the room!

Also, many hotels use a chemical wash (as do most banquet and restaurant facilities; so remember to use your napkin to wipe the glass before wine or water is poured into it!) in order to get that spotless finish on the glasses. You do ***not*** want to ingest those chemicals.

I have also seen maids who have colds moving the glasses (in order to clean under them). Heaven only knows what or who touches those glasses. Save yourself from infection, and tell housekeeping not to touch any of your room's glasses. The maids will be happy because it saves them work. It is wise to place a tissue over the top of your glasses and anchor it with a comb, toothbrush, or pen. This is always a signal for "Do Not Touch". Then it is usually left alone.

FOOD STORE / SUPERMARKET / ANY STORE CHECKOUT: BEWARE OF GERMS

Too often one finds that a **cashier** checking you out **has a cold** or a cough. They do not even bother to hide it while they sniffle and cough over your purchase and pick each item up to bag it with their germy fingers. Do not hesitate to protect your health and pleasantly tell the cashier, "Oh, I see that you don't feel well. Let me do the packing." If it becomes necessary, just tell them that you worry about germs and do not want their fingers on your food or other items.

TEA and LOOSE LEAF TEA

Tea is a healthful and wonderful beverage with wide variety. For those who do not use loose leaf tea, please try it. It is the healthiest form of tea (which I mention, because with tea bags, it is difficult to know exactly what grade is the leaf [a bag could actually contain lowest grades called fannings or dust] AND of what ingredients the <u>bag</u> is made [one must worry about bleaches, chemicals, and other components]), and if one buys the highest grade loose tea, the taste is sublime. All that one needs is a pot for brewing and a strainer.

Yes, it is more work than a tea bag; however, **everything that you do to improve your health is not work but <u>effort</u>! It takes effort to stay healthy into one's nineties, and every little improvement contributes to that health.**

I have a long knowledge of tea (one could say that I am *steeped* in it [enjoy a chuckle; it is good for one's health]) and, over the years, have advised private restaurants regarding tea menus. A friend of mine was a lifetime friend of King Juan Carlos of Spain, who appreciated my heartfelt knowledge and my ability to identify a tea by its aroma. "It is not to be learned but must be inborn" as King Juan Carlos once complimented me at a private luncheon.

HOW TO PREPARE TEA

I recommend a full half teaspoon of loose tea per mug of water; put tea leaves into a glass or china pot for brewing, which I place on a metal warming implement over a gas burner (light very low). Boil the exact amount of water in another pot, and pour it over the middle mound of those leaves. I prefer steeping for six (and sometimes seven) minutes. Place the strainer (or lacking a strainer, even a paper towel) over the cup, and pour in the exquisite tea. One can always brew stronger or lighter teas to your taste.

Personally, I buy loose tea from Pacific Place in Honolulu; NK in Stockholm, Sweden; Te & Kaffi in Reykjavik, Iceland; and McNulty's in Greenwich Village, New York City.

Pacific Place is a Hawaii treasure. Lynette Jee is the founder and owner. I first tasted teas from Pacific Place when staying at the Halekulani Hotel in Honolulu. Lynette travels to tea auctions and sells top-grade teas, and deluxe hotels as well as Neiman Marcus are her clients. May I suggest some of my favorites: **Magnolia Oolong** (this is the *most* extraordinary oolong that one can enjoy—soft, fragrant, delicate), **Passion for Hawaii** (a Ceylon tea with passion fruit nectar, papaya, and pineapple fruit—luscious and deep), two superb **Darjeeling** (a Puttabong Estates First Flush and also a robust Second Flush), the finest **Pineapple Coconut Rooibos** that I ever tasted, and the best **organic peppermint** one could want. There are many more to view **at www.thepacificplace.com**. Many people enjoy tea black, while I use whole goat milk or cream in all except rooibos. Yes, I put cream in Magnolia Oolong!

For those who enjoy a **perfect decaffeinated tea, Passion for Hawaii Decaffeinated** from Pacific Place is extraordinary! The aroma and rich taste provide a tea that is unique to decaffeinated teas!

Te & Kaffi in Iceland is also an absolute gem! I found this family treasure, located on Laugavegur, on my first visit when strolling this main, historic shopping street (in Reykjavík) which is home to some of the most exclusive stores. Reykjavik is a most cosmopolitan, sophisticated city with superb restaurants. Te & Kaffi on Laugavegur has both a tea and coffee shop and a coffeehouse, and there are nine other locations in Iceland. Founded and owned by the wonderful Sigmundur Dýrfjörð and his charming wife, Berglind Guðbrandsdóttir, they sell many loose leaf teas of highest grades, coffee, and confections. View everything at **http://www.teogkaffi.is**. I particularly enjoy their **perfect Yunnan** (I have never found Yunnan this good anywhere else), several luscious **Darjeeling**, **Apricot**, sublime **Mango**, and one of the most superb teas: **extraordinary Solber** (black currant). One can telephone and order or e-mail.

There many teas that I buy from **NK Kaffe & Tehandel (www.nk.se)**. The easiest way to communicate is to telephone them, speak with one of the ladies in the tea salon, and then order from her by e-mail. Some of my favorites are **Sommarblandning, Elderflower, Kaktusblom,** and **Svarta Jordgubb Flader** (which is strawberry elderflower). These teas are unique and unbelievable.

McNulty's in Greenwich Village (New York City) is there since 1895 and was honored on Sunday, January 19, 2014 with a wonderful article in *The New York Times*. What a perfect establishment for buying teas and coffees as you enter this family business—owned by Wing Wong and his son David Wong—on Christopher Street in the heart of Manhattan's Greenwich Village (**www.mcnultys.com**). The aromas of teas and coffees are divine. Again, there are *many* loose teas, but I also recommend the **passion fruit** and the **black currant**, both fragrant and delicious, as well as the unique **Tanzania Luponde**. I have known David and his dad for over three decades. McNulty's is ageless!

CAROLE LYNN STEINER

WASHING FRUITS AND VEGETABLES:
NEVER Antibacterial Soaps or Wipes

The concerns today over eating clean and safe foods are legion. Washing produce is critical. Wash fruits (including melons) with a soapy sponge (Ivory soap or with Omega Nutrition's liquid soap), rinse them thoroughly, and then soak them in a pot (one-quart size or whatever size suits the produce) of mild warm water with four drops of **NutriBiotic Grapefruit Seed Extract** *stirred* in. Soak for ten minutes. Do not rinse.

With vegetables, put them in a big pot or container and rinse extremely well. Then put some liquid soap (***not*** antibacterial!) into the water and again rinse thoroughly. Once the soap is gone, make a pot of tepid water with the grapefruit seed extract (four drops in one quart of water [stir the drops with your hand or a spoon]), and soak for ten minutes.

The grapefruit seed extract is antibacterial and can be protective. Since GSE is also edible, you do ***not*** wash it off the produce. Just let the produce air-dry on a clean terry towel. The GSE will keep the produce fresh longer, including in the refrigerator.

WHY did I write (above) "not antibacterial" soap? Because you do not want those poisonous chemicals on your food and, even worse, **leaching into the produce**. While NutriBiotic Grapefruit Seed Extract is antibacterial, it is also edible. **Antibacterial soap is not edible. It is poison.** Note that those antibacterial wipes and cleansers are loaded with chemicals, which, entering the bloodstream, are toxic! **Stop** constantly using them as the active ingredient may be linked to endocrine disruption and cancer. It can also disrupt proper thyroid functioning. Children's hands should ***not*** be wiped with them, because children put their hands to their mouths all the time, and this product is toxic if ingested.

Remember, washing hands with regular soap for thirty seconds is just as good!

PILLOWS AND TEDDY BEARS
Eliminate Dust Mites Using Cold Air

Dust mites live inside pillows and fluffy teddy bears and other stuffed toys. Cold kills them. Some references indicate that seventy degrees Fahrenheit and under while others say fifty and under would be the temperature at which mites can be killed. I believe that the colder the more effective for killing them. Keep your home cool and dry, because those mites also like humidity.

Personal Note: Almost every cold weather morning (starting in autumn) I put our pillows into two big shopping bags and place them out on the terrace. It is sunny as well as nice and cold there. I leave them for ten minutes sometimes but usually for a few hours.

For those without an outside area, turn on the air-conditioner in your smallest room, set it very cold, and allow the pillows and stuffed animals to stay in that cold for an hour or longer.

WATERING PLANTS, GARDENING WITH HYDROGEN PEROXIDE!

Yes, indeed! That inexpensive bottle of 3 percent hydrogen peroxide can enhance plants and gardens.

When the garden is watered by rain, there is a small amount of hydrogen peroxide in the water. It is part of the earth's cleaning system. Using a half cup 3 percent hydrogen peroxide to a gallon of tepid water for watering plants will green them, perk up sick plants, and prevent or kill molds and fungal infections. Never overuse this. More is not better. I also suggest using this one week and taking the next week off. Adjust the amount according to how much water is in a watering can.

The tap water normally used for watering plants does not contain hydrogen peroxide, but it can be added to enrich the water. Peroxide helps maintain healthy soil and allows roots to breathe better. Peroxide can be used as plant food for any type of indoor as well as outdoor plants. Remember to wash off any peroxide that gets onto your skin. It is not harmful; it is just unnecessary.

As a foliage pest spray, mix equal amounts of 3 percent hydrogen peroxide and distilled water. Spray once a week or after it rains on both the tops and undersides of leaves. This will both treat current and prevent further infestation.

CHRISTMAS TREES: Here is one method for keeping one's Christmas tree nice and fresh: use 3 percent hydrogen peroxide! **Hydrogen peroxide** (so inexpensive and available at all drugstores) works well to **keep the water clear of bacteria** and can **provide more oxygen to the tree cells, which will keep the tree fresh and green longer**. Mix one part hydrogen peroxide to about four parts water and add to the reservoir that holds the tree. Of course, only water the tree when the lights are shut off.

STRESS

You do not even realize (sometimes) that you have it! There are *symptoms*.

I was only twenty-two years old but was suffering—and quite suddenly—from **ringing in the ears**. So on this exquisite, sunny June day, I was walking north on Park Avenue in Manhattan to see my father's cousin Dr. Samuel Rosen. Dr. Sam (as the family called this world-renowned doctor who gained global fame from developing the Rosen stapes operation to restore hearing) was a preeminent ear surgeon and had developed operations to cure certain forms of deafness. The singer Johnnie Ray was treated by Dr. Sam. He travelled the world teaching his delicate operation, was always the guest of the head of state, and donated operating rooms to the hospitals where he taught. He passed away in Beijing (on a trip with his wife, Helen), and he is the only foreigner for whom a state funeral was ever given in China.

I was very worried about my hearing when I called him, and Sam had said, "Come on in." He examined me and had hearing tests administered, after which we sat down in his manly, clubby office. He quietly looked at me and said, "Now tell me what is bothering you." I looked blank. He said, "What is wrong? What is upsetting you?" I was quiet for a moment and then said, "Nothing. Really nothing, Sam."

And Sam said what I have remembered all my life, "Well, sweetheart, whenever what is <u>not</u> bothering you goes away, so will the ringing in your ears!"

He was SO right! It was my first lesson in something being a *symptom* and not the disease. I was under terrible stress. My husband wanted us to move quite a distance away, and there were other problems. While I considered this stress part of life and normal, my body did not.

About a month later, all my personal problems were happily resolved, and, you know it, the ringing in my ears disappeared.

I have always blessed and remembered dear Dr. Sam. He had reassured me, calmed me as he patted my hand while we talked, and with a big hug and kiss good-bye, I left his office with no worry.

Stress can manifest itself through many symptoms. Ringing in the ears, itching in the middle of the back between the shoulder blades (especially from adrenal burnout or fatigue)—these are ***symptoms****.* **The body is alerting you.** Never treat a symptom. Always treat the cause.

Supplements: When I am under huge stress, I take Standard Process Drenamin (three tablets three times daily), which promotes healthy adrenal gland function. I take a significant group of supplements, and Drenamin is very helpful when I need to focus on the adrenal gland. The symptom that I get is itching in the middle of the back. It stops within minutes of taking Drenamin.

FULL-SPECTRUM LIGHTBULBS—NATURAL LIGHTING

Lighting as one gets it from the sun is the best lighting for reading and work. I have introduced this to a number of **doctors**. After seeing their exhausted red eyes after a day of work, I explain that full-spectrum lighting will protect their eyes as well as—importantly—give them better, clearer vision of their patients. The same is true for one in an **office**. After a long day, poor lighting shows in **strained eyes.** A Verilux lamp with a full-spectrum bulb also provides beneficial natural light on one's computer monitor.

I have bought **Verilux** bulbs for years in the frosted 60 watt, 100 watt, three-way including 150 watt, and candelabra (for chandeliers) for both my **home and office**. If you have latitude over what lights can be used in your office, please do use **full-spectrum** lighting. Even where I have overhead fluorescent lights in the office, I replace them with natural **full-spectrum** lighting. This is available from Verilux (various sales throughout the year) and from **Lowe's** and **Home Depot**. Compare prices when buying, and watch for sales. **NOTE**: Under a new US law, our wonderful lightbulbs are being replaced with bulbs which contain mercury and do not produce light as we knew it. Currently, I am buying many 60 and 150 watt bulbs and storing them.

PROOF THAT CONSISTENT DIET AND SUPPLEMENTS WORK

This past June, my eye doctor said that I am THE ONLY PATIENT HE EVER HAD WHOSE **PRESCRIPTION (for nearsightedness) GOT BETTER OVER THE YEARS,** and **I NOW HAVE NO ASTIGMATISM.** My reading vision has always been perfect!

I became nearsighted at age seventeen and needed a prescription for distance vision. I also had mild astigmatism. Once I took control of my health (see article "Cervical Dysplasia") and some years passed, suddenly my eye doctor found that my distance vision had improved and my astigmatism had lessened.

This past June, though, he was really amazed. My **distance vision was even better** AND there was **no more** astigmatism. The doctor said, "Carole, I really think I'm going to take whatever **supplements** you do! I never saw such progress!"

Personal Note: I also believe that my inverting on the slant board (of my Total Gym) increased blood flow to my head, which nourished my eyes and brain. (See "Hang Upside Down").

CERVICAL DYSPLASIA
What Started Carole Lynn on the Road to Natural Health Care?

I placed this article toward the end, thinking, *This will now sum up for you, dear reader, the reasons for the path taken by my life in following natural health care.* **How and why did *I* start to take control of my own health? It was, indeed, to save my own life.**

I had returned from a business trip in Southeast Asia. It was 7:30 am on a gorgeous September morning, and I was rushing along Central Park South for a breakfast meeting in the Edwardian Room of the Plaza Hotel with the ambassador to the United States from Thailand. I had just passed the St. Moritz Hotel (now the Ritz-Carlton) when my high heel (note: I *now* wear nice-looking flats for walking and rushing) sank into a crack, and I was plummeting face forward to the ground. I dropped my briefcase and purse as I threw my arms up to protect my face. Hence, I hit the ground chest first. I can still hear the gasping of business people on the sidewalk and murmurings; "Ohhh, she's falling" and "Catch her . . . catch her" and "This is bad." I had the air completely knocked out of me, so I could not move or talk. One gentleman knelt down and said, "Miss, I have your pocketbook," while another gentleman said, "I have your briefcase and shoes. Don't worry."

Suddenly, kneeling next to me and patting my back was a big, handsome policeman. He had driven his patrol car partially up on the sidewalk and was murmuring, "You had a very bad fall. I saw the whole thing. Don't worry. I called an ambulance." Hearing that, I turned my head, looked in his eyes (he *was* handsome), and just shook my head no. He said, "No?" and I shook no. He was also smart! "Ah," he said, "you had the air knocked out of you." I smiled and nodded.

Finally, I could get a few words out. Only a couple of minutes had passed, but it seemed like an hour that I was lying there in my new winter-white wool suit. The doorman of the apartment building said, "Why don't you help the young lady in here. She can sit down." The policeman scooped me up, the other kind gentlemen brought my belongings, and I pulled myself together in the lobby. After all, I had a breakfast meeting to get to despite a hole in the hem of my new suit.

Two days passed, and I was concerned because my heart was still racing. It just was not pumping smoothly. At the time, I was a junior trustee at the Hospital for Joint Diseases (now part of NYU Langone Medical Center), and I called the director of the hospital. He immediately told me that I would see "our fantastic internist", and I went right downtown to the hospital. This excellent doctor checked all the usual things and also gave me an EKG and an EEG. **HERE COMES THE BEGINNING.** He then said, "Shall I also do a Pap smear?" I said, "Well, our old family doctor—who is on vacation—always does that, but sure, why not." Good thing!

Three days passed, and the doctor called me. He was somewhat breathless as he said, "You're fine. You're fine. You had a very bad fall, but you'll be fine. But you have a funny Pap smear!" I said, "Funny ha-ha, or funny peculiar?" He went on, "There are five classes of Pap smears: class 1 is perfect, class 5 is cancer, and you have class 2." I asked, "Why?" and he said that cells were not forming correctly and asked, "Do you know a good OB-GYN doctor?" Actually, I did. This doctor was a big name at that time, and the internist was very happy and knew of his reputation.

First, I called our old family doctor, who was now home from vacation, and told him what had transpired. He said, "Oh, sweetheart, a class 2 Pap smear is no big deal. Most women are walking around with that. You've had that for over a year. And there is nothing you can do about it anyway." So much for that old doctor!

That night, I sat down with my mother, father, and my boyfriend and discussed this thing called cervical dysplasia. My mother was going to call friends and ask if anyone had it. The next day I started calling women's groups. NOW (National Organization for Women) sent me excellent literature and, with a donation from me, sent a book. **Slowly I started learning about cells that become dysplastic; they fail to** mature properly. This can develop into cancer. But I did not yet know why, and no one writing about this seemed to know why.

I had an appointment with the OB-GYN doctor, who then said, "This is easy to treat. We 'go in' and freeze the dysplastic cells [with a gas]. They freeze and fall off." This was called cryosurgery. Well, they may have frozen and fallen; however, the new cells were no better than the old. **Something was causing this, and I wanted to know what it was!**

I assembled a list of thirteen doctors who were heads of OB-GYN departments at the largest medical centers in the metropolitan area of New York City, and I had appointments to see every one of them over the next two months. Meanwhile, I stopped working and secreted myself in the medical library at the Hospital for Joint Diseases. **I pulled up microfilm and microfiche articles on cervical dysplasia and started learning that some doctors around the world were reversing this with vitamins!**

So I bought books on supplements (*see Mybyble article* "Learn")—some of them several hundred pages (I took copious notes)—and started learning the value of supplements to the body and the *symptoms* that show deficiencies in the body.

Dysplastic cells are a symptom showing that the body is being deprived of certain nutrients. I read vast numbers of medical research articles in the hospital's medical library and found doctors using nutrients to reverse this in the Karolinska Institutet in Stockholm and the National Institutes of Health in Australia and New Zealand and Bethesda, Maryland, and also the University of Alabama Medical Center in Birmingham and the University of Arizona Medical Center in Scottsdale.

I got telephone numbers and called every one of them! Each doctor was amazed that I had tracked him down and all but one were delighted to speak with me about their research. The two major nutrients being used were folate and vitamin A. They discussed doses with me (as written in their research papers) and length of time for success. Indeed, **these doctors believed that dysplastic cells are a symptom of deficiencies in either vitamin A or folate.**

The one snippy doctor, lo and behold, was from a significant medical center in my own country. The funny thing is that having read his research, I also found an article that misquoted the dose about which he reported. The misquote indicated a dose thousands of times greater than what should have been stated, because it stated milligrams instead of micrograms. When I got him on the telephone, he snapped at me, "Who are you? How did you get this number?" Very fresh. I explained who I was, what I had been doing, and how I reached him. He said, "Well! You don't expect me to discuss my research with *you*, do you?" I told him the names of some of the biggest research scientists in the world, including Dr. Linus Pauling and Dr. Ewan Cameron, who had spoken with me, and then I asked him if, lacking any other conversation with me, he would like to know in what article he had been egregiously misquoted (which could lead to people's deaths and law suits). He was shocked. He said, "*I* was misquoted? Where? What did they say?" I told him. He actually then thanked me and then did discuss his successful research using folate.

I started developing a supplement protocol with folate and vitamin A, slowly adding other nutrients as I researched them and learned. I took **400 mcg of folate two times daily before meals and 10,000 IUs of vitamin A two times daily with meals. Fats are needed in the stomach for proper digestion, and I believe in spacing out the taking of supplements in order to maximize absorption. I also took 500 mg of vitamin C four times daily**.

Now back to those thirteen OB-GYN doctors and my appointments. I went to every appointment, and with each one, they wanted me to sign a consent form that if the doctor looked inside me and performed any surgery or removal, they had my approval. Well, they did not—and I would not sign any form permitting outpatient surgery. I explained that I still had my tonsils and every other part of my body, I had never been operated on, I had not yet had children, I had never broken a bone, and I had no interest in anyone doing any procedure without first consulting with me!

Each doctor took a look, and each thought that additional cryosurgery might work. I already knew otherwise. **Repeating a failed treatment is not, in my opinion, valid!** I did ask each of them about vitamins for reversing cervical dysplasia and was told "Impossible". I told them about the research by medical doctors that proved it, and not one of these doctors cared.

Here is a **funny** story. Only one of these thirteen top doctors was a woman. The medical director of Joint Diseases had introduced her to me, and I called her for an appointment. She spoke with me, we discussed the condition, set a date, and then I gently asked, "By the way, doctor, do you know about all the research showing certain vitamins reverse cervical dysplasia?" Well, she exploded and cursed me out like I had never heard before, practically spitting these exact words through the telephone: "Vitamins! F——ing vitamins! If another f——ing person asks me another f——ing question about vitamins for ANYthing, I will throw that f——ing person out my office window. And let me tell you that I am on the fourth floor of the building!" I quietly replied, "You know, doctor, let's just cancel that appointment," and I gently hung up the telephone. I then called the medical director who had introduced her, told him about this, and said, "I suggest that she may not be the most reliable source for treatment for ANYone for ANYthing."

The thirteenth doctor was the best in that I finally got an informative description of dysplasia, what causes it, and that vitamins "might help."

This doctor was head of OB-GYN at one of the largest New York medical centers outside of Manhattan. He was not the usual doctor one expects. He wore an open-necked shirt, gold chains, and was (to use a word of that time) quite mod. Again, I refused to sign any form for outpatient surgery. Once he had examined me, we met in his office to talk, and it was indeed illuminating.

He described the condition (and my class 2) and explained that these cells, which fail to form and *mature correctly,* are because something has interfered with their development. "Yes," he posited, "I can understand the vitamin connection." Then he threw me with "**I can tell you more about this than most other doctors, because I am the cofounder of the birth control pill.** There is no question but that the pill eats up vitamins that you take in from your food, and I can see that they should be supplemented. But there is something else. I can objectively tell this to you because I am a man [so it is not a woman blaming a man]. The problem with the pill is that it has stopped people from using condoms, and the **most allergenic substance that a woman can put into her body is sperm!**" My eyes popped! "Sperm is meant for creating life and not for inserting into the body over and over just for sex. And multiple sex partners increase the occurrence of dysplasia. Sperm from different sources disrupts the internal lining and functioning of the cervix. So if your partner cares about you—and your health—he will use a condom."

I sat there wide-eyed as he nodded. It was totally logical and explained much about the condition's development for so many women, especially with the birth control pill.

That night, I sat down with my parents and boyfriend. We decided: I look healthy; I am healthy. I am learning about what I can do to treat this condition. I am not having anyone cut me open. Later, my boyfriend (who had been with me at the conference with this final doctor) immediately said, "Let's go buy condoms." And we did.

First thing, I revised my diet. I had always loved fruit and raw vegetables, but now I increased them tremendously: fruit first thing in the morning (read article "Food Combining") and vegetables before dinner. I reduced my wine intake. Most of all, **I kept reading and learning, and I took control of my health.**

I added nutrient supplements one by one as I read how each could enhance my health. I maintained my continuous reading about supplements and refined my protocol as necessary. It was a lengthy process initially and took three years to develop my program.

And then it happened. I opened *The New York Times* one morning and found an article about a doctor at a prestigious College of Medicine finding that he could **reverse cervical dysplasia with vitamin C!** I almost fell off my chair. I immediately got the telephone number, called, asked for this doctor's office, and reached his secretary. (In those days, one did not deal with robots answering calls at major numbers. You reached an operator who would put you through to your party!) I told this lovely woman my story, and she said, "Do you mean to tell me that after you had a class 2 Pap smear, you started supplement and diet therapy, and you have not seen a doctor in three years?" "Yes, exactly." "Well," she exclaimed, "the doctor is head of cancer research and does not usually see patients, but I bet he'll want to see you!" She took my number.

In about fifteen minutes, she called me back and asked if I could come to the office the next day. He was a wonderful man. We hit it off right away. He listened to my story and said, "I tell you what. I believe in people taking vitamins. If I examine you and find that you are now OK, you have to promise to speak at some of my fund-raising meetings. All these business leaders are always telling me, 'Oh, I'm too busy to take vitamins. I can't be bothered.' Well, **if you could rearrange your life in order to save it,** other people should hear your story and use vitamins to take care of their health too."

We shook hands. It was a deal. He examined me, did a Pap smear, and called me a few days later. My test was now class 1! Perfect. Believe me, I was grateful and relieved.

At that time, I increased the vitamin C for my supplements to 1,000 mg three times (and even four times) daily; however, currently I use Standard Process (SP) A-C-P and sometimes SP Collagen C. The dose for A-C-P sounds considerably less than when one hears about 500 mg three or more times daily, because SP products are whole food-based, and it takes smaller doses to be effective. Of course, I took and still take a folate supplement before breakfast, as well as vitamin A. See article "Fish Oil and Vitamin A". See the "Source List" for product information.

I always made (and still do) copious notes during and after telephone calls and meetings. Hence, my detailed recall. Then, too, I have repeated this story so many times over the years and have helped so many women.

OZONE THERAPY: There is one treatment that must be shared with you. I first learned about it from a woman I met who swam the English Channel. She related that at one time, her (female) doctor told her that she had a class 3 Pap smear. This is a precancerous state that needs attention. Her doctor wanted to cut her open, but this woman decided to try a diet change, vitamins, and **ozone therapy!**

She purchased an ozone machine in order to introduce ozone through her vagina into the cervix. Six months went by, and she went back to that doctor for another Pap smear. The doctor refused. She said, "We already did that. You need surgery." My friend said, "I have been using natural treatments, and I think I may be better. Why not check?" The doctor was furious, and finally my friend went to another doctor. Her new Pap smear was class 1. Perfect. She stopped back at the original doctor's office in order to tell her, and the doctor could not care less. My friend said, "Don't you want to know what I did so you could help other women?" The doctor asked her nurse to "show this woman out".

I know of a few other women who **used ozone generators for vaginal insufflation for mild cervical dysplasia for thirty minutes daily for two months. Their dysplasia was gone.**

There is significant information on ozone therapy online.

WE HAVE NOW COVERED HEALTH AND LIFESTYLE TIPS.
WE NOW CONSIDER:
AS PRECIOUS AS HEALTH IS YOUR WEALTH.

INVESTING, MARGIN

I have spoken on Bloomberg Radio, television, and other networks numerous times, and these three presentations on Bloomberg garnered excellent audience response.

My grandfather and father told me that those who margin heavily over the course of their lifetimes would be wiped out three times. In watching investor accounts over many years as a broker holding several licenses, that seems to be accurate. I have heard horror stories over the losses as well as the misadvice given to investors by brokers and also by friends.

MYBYBLE

There are several points that help to clarify this topic:

1. The safest equity investing is in a cash account fully owned by <u>you</u> (and in <u>your</u> name, not "house" name). This is also the most flexible type of account because you can sell individual positions and not be locked into a fund.

2. If one margins, do not margin more than you have cash to cover. Never margin to the hilt.

3. Do not margin when the market is high and raging upward. Any retrenchment (from any bad news) will catch you.

4. If one is intent upon margining, the ideal time is when the market is at rock bottom: when everyone is sighing, when New York Stock Exchange volume is low, when all the good companies (large cap, cash rich) are ridiculously low—especially if the market slide has gone on for twelve or more months—and when PE ratios are realistic. **THESE POINTS ARE INVALUABLE**. In fact, I have lived through such markets. A market crash is always incvitable. Some incomprehensible bad news—such as the attack of September 11—is bound to come. That is when one can margin, but again, *only* if you have cash to cover. It is almost inevitable that if someone margins and has no cash to cover, **that** is when the market will plummet more.

5. If the market is going up, consider placing stop-loss orders at 10 percent beneath current prices in order to protect yourself from a terrible backslide. Should the stock price go down well below the price at which you get out, you can always buy it back if the fundamentals are sound. Otherwise, one can watch for a worthwhile buy of another company that has been beaten down.

CAROLE LYNN STEINER

THE EXTENDED LIFESPAN, and ARE YOU PREPARED FOR IT FINANCIALLY?

This was the title of the biggest program that I presented on Bloomberg Radio in 2000. At that time, no one had addressed this critical topic. The audience, though, was waiting for just such help. My Bloomberg producer told me that the program broke the record for call-ins. By the time that I left the Bloomberg studio on upper Park Avenue and got down to my Wall Street office, my producer was calling me in order to tell me that there was a record call-in and that everyone wanted my telephone number. He said, "They are all saying that they want the number for 'that girl'!" It was quite a day.

I discussed investing at different stages of life. I talked about safety, diversity, flexibility, and timing.

Diversity comes from holding stocks in different industries or areas. If one holds bonds, one wants them in diverse communities or corporations.

Flexibility comes from owning your own individual positions and not holding funds. Flexibility allows the sale of any single position as opposed to being in a fund where the entire fund must be liquidated. Flexibility also relates to taxes. If one is in a fund, one is liable for any taxes accrued by the fund manager, as positions—throughout the year—are bought and sold and thereby, at times, costing the investor tax dollars even though one has not liquidated the fund.

Timing was discussed in relation to a down market as well as an up market. I also melded flexibility with timing, because owning individual positions allows one to sell at the very moment that one desires an execution, whereas with certain funds, one cannot always get an immediate execution.

Safety is involved with all these topics: investing cautiously, thinking through any moves, doing what is appropriate for you and the monetary funds that you have or will have, buying stocks of well-known, large-cap companies and industries that have a history as well as a future, and never being pressured into buying or selling.

I spoke at length (on Bloomberg) having been allowed a longer segment than the usual programs due to the unique importance of the topic. Included in the presentation was information on interviewing a prospective investment advisor and also when (if ever) to margin the account. *Mybyble* has two articles on these topics bookending this article.

INVESTING: HOW TO INTERVIEW AN INVESTMENT ADVISOR

The Broker

For most people, **the most important concerns in life are family, health, and finances. You would not entrust your family or your health to someone who is inept, uneducated, or uncaring, nor should you so sacrifice your money.**

In interviewing prospective advisors (yes, *interview* them), ask the following questions: Is your record clean? How long have you been registered? Where did you get your training? (A three-week crash course for a former messenger, clerk, or salesman [from another field] is not sufficient to produce an experienced advisor.) What stocks do you own and how long have you owned them? Did your parents and grandparents invest? Were you brought up hearing conversations about investing?

I myself would not want anyone looking after my finances who either did not have more than I have—or at least as much—or have a substantial amount invested.

Also inquire: How many **down** cycles have you lived through? Have you lost your own money? I would not want any advisor who has not experienced at least two down cycles in the market and who has not lost money of his/her own. The person who has not lost money has no knowledge of what such a loss means and no realization of how devastating it can be. *That* advisor is not in an experienced position to fully protect a client.

Your intuition is generally correct. If someone seems not right for you or not meshed with your thinking, go on to someone else. One cannot have a wild speculator giving you hot tips and heart failure if you are basically a safety-oriented conservative at heart.

The Portfolio

A balanced portfolio is crucial. Please see the two *Mybyble* articles "Margin" and "The Extended Lifespan, and Are You Prepared for It Financially?" I spoke on these topics on television and radio, and the two articles provide details.

SOURCE LIST—Assembled by Category and Not Alphabetically

I am very careful to refer to exactly what products *I* have used. Success surely depends upon a pure product containing healthy attributes. Other products vary in their ingredients as well as their processing. It took years for me to research and find the products to which I refer, and I continuously and diligently read medical research, health newsletters, and articles that contribute to this complete and always growing knowledge base. It is also critical that a company can be telephoned and that a customer can speak with a professional representative and get answers to questions. I only buy from suppliers that are consistent, reliable, accurate, responsive, and well priced.

Do NOT refrigerate coconut oils, emu oil, apple cider vinegar, or honey. They are stable at room temperature and have a long shelf life. Keep other supplements in a cool, dry cabinet or closet.

Note that many of the products come in various sizes. Go online to view and price them.

Omega Nutrition, www.omeganutrition.com, 800-661-3529.
Products (remember for gifts):
- **Organic *Virgin* Coconut Oil** (which I use on face, scalp, freckles; bread, toast along with Organic Valley Cultured Butter)
- **Organic Coconut Oil** (which I use on pasta [along with high-lignan flax oil and a hefty sprinkle of **Cold-Milled Flax Seeds**]; greasing and basting chickens, turkeys, potatoes; scrambled eggs [coconut oil on pan before scrambling]; diminishing freckles)
- **Organic Apple Cider Vinegar** Unfiltered, Unpasteurized, with "the mother"
- **Flax oil** (choose either plain or high lignan; this must be refrigerated; extra bottles can be frozen)
- **Cold-Milled Flax Seeds** (must be refrigerated; extra canisters can be frozen)
- Two other products: Natural **Bar Soap and Liquid Soap**

(Most Omega Nutrition products come in more than one size.)

Thunder Ridge Emu Oil, www.thunderridgeemu.com, 800-457-0617. Good gift.

Selina Naturally, www.selinanaturally.com, 800-867-7258.
Products: **Celtic Sea Salt** (both light grey [chunky] and fine). Be sure to become a member and get special prices. View website for all products. Remember for gifts.

Good-Gums, www.good-gums.com, 888-693-0333.

Probiotics from **Mt. Capra: Caprabiotics Plus+** (120 count), 800-574-1961. This product must be either refrigerated or kept in the freezer. I put a dozen capsules in a small bottle in the refrigerator while keeping the larger bottle in the freezer. Mt. Capra also has other probiotics that do not need refrigeration.

GUM PerioBalance from Sunstar Americas Inc (in the US), 888-777-3101, www.sunstaramericas.com. Special price and free shipping when buying three boxes instead of one.

Future Sticks, www.futuresticks.com. Currently, use special code FS1 for a discount. Telephone 816-600-8737. The permanent, safe chopstick. Great gift.

Floss Sticks: Plackers Gentle Fine (for tight teeth) Dental Flossers. Walgreens, www.walgreens.com.

Thayers Slippery Elm Lozenges available at Swanson, Vitacost, Vitamin Shoppe, Health Nuts. Varying size containers and prices. Lowest prices usually at Swanson and Vitacost.

Douglas Laboratories: All the products from Douglas Labs mentioned in the digestives article are available from health-care professionals. View www.douglaslabs.com in order to get item numbers (for the size that you want to order) or communicate with the company. Products:

- **Osteo-guard (calcium:** #OSG—120 count)
- **Amino-Mag (magnesium:** #MAG—100 count)
- **Vitamin D3** (#83007-100 count)

- **Betaine Plus** (#80106-250 count)
- **Lipanase** (#LPN—90 count)
- **Vegetarian Enzymes** (#7048-120 count)
- **Horsetail Grass Max-V** (Item #77350. Standardized 7% silica [10% silicic acid] 60 capsules. Take before **injections** [for example, for two days prior to Juvéderm for wrinkles] to help prevent excessive bleeding.)

The Vitamin Shoppe, www.vitaminshoppe.com, 866-293-3367. Ask them to make you a Vitamin Shoppe member. You will get a number linked to your account, and at the end of every year, you will receive a **monetary gift certificate** based upon a percentage of what you spent. This certificate is for use in the store. **SALES**: There are sales throughout the year. Sign up for e-mails in order to be kept informed. Products:
- **NutriBiotic Grapefruit Seed Extract** (2 oz. bottle with eyedropper top; item NQ-2001)
- VS brand **High Gamma E** (400 IU; item VS-1888)
- VS brand **Milk Thistle Extract** (175 mg; item VS-1725)

I have only found these last two products at Vitamin Shoppe with these exact ingredients and dosages. Note that there are smaller count bottles. **NutriBiotic GSE** is also available directly from www.nutribiotic.com, and there are sales during the year (800-225-4345).

Swanson, www.swansonvitamins.com, 800-437-4148.
Vitacost, www.vitacost.com, 800-381-0759.
Puritan's Pride, www.puritan.com, 800-645-1030.
Puritan's products:
- **Glycerin soap** (four bars per pack, #1560)
- **Echinacea** (#5633, also one larger size)
- **Pau d'Arco** (#5634)
- **Charcoal** 260 mg (4 grains, #3680)
- **Alfalfa** (#046291) 10 grain/650 mg
- **Bee Propolis** 500 mg in several-size bottles. Also, **Swanson** (#SW324) 550 mg

Kyolic Garlic Formula 100 Discounted at Swanson and Vitacost. There are three sizes: 100, 200, and 300 capsules. The 200 and 300 count are the best values.

SWANSON, VITACOST, AND PURITAN'S PRIDE HAVE SALES ALL YEAR ROUND, SPECIAL DEALS, AND EXCELLENT CUSTOMER SERVICE. Sign up for e-mails in order to be informed.

Maca Organic Powder #SWF122 (Swanson). Capsules also available.
Vitex Agnus-Castus Chaste Berry #NSI3006038 (Vitacost). Liquid drops also available.

Olive Leaf Extract (#SWH158 = 60 count; #SWH159 = 120 count) and **Prickly Pear Cactus Opuntia** (#SW543). Both from Swanson.

Source Natural Vitamin A 10,000 IU tablets. From Swanson or Vitacost.
Selenium L-Selenomethionine from Swanson (#SW545), 300 capsules, 100 mcg.
L-Tryptophan TryptoPure from Swanson (#SWU372), 90 capsules, 500 mg.
Suntheanine L-Theanine from Swanson (#SWU110) 60 capsules, 100 mg.
Folate 5-Methyltetrahydrofolic Acid from Swanson (#SWU758) 400 mcg.
PABA from Swanson (#SW1367), 120 *capsules*, 500 mg. *Tablets* are available from Puritan's Pride (#2920).
L-OptiZinc (#NSI 3001095) from Vitacost, 200 capsules, 30 mg.

Mayumi Squalane (2.17 fl. oz.): I buy this from either Swanson or Vitacost.
Desert Essence Organic Jojoba Oil (4 fl. oz.): I buy from Swanson or Vitacost.
Nivea Creme bought from CVS (www.cvs.com) and Walgreens (www.walgreens.com).
Wet n' Wild Cover Stick as well as nail polish and lipsticks. Bought from CVS and Walgreens.

Both **JCPenney** (www.jcpenney.com) and **T.J. Maxx** (www.Tjmax.com) often sell discounted very **soft terry washcloths and towels.** They are usually Egyptian cotton and made in Portugal or Colombia. Of course, they can be bought at full price in many stores.

Gymnasium: Total Gym, www.totalgym.com, 800-541-4900. Thirty years ago, I bought the WestBend Gymnasium. Today, the closest to my gym is from Total Gym. View the website and see the different models. During the year, they have sales. Sign up for e-mails. One can also go to any exercise equipment store (and research online) in order to compare prices as well as models. I use my gym to lie upside down as well as to exercise my arms by pulling myself both backward and forward.

Angled slant pad: Available in many exercise equipment stores and discount stores.

Minitrampoline (rebounder): I have mostly bought my rebounders from Walmart (www.walmart.com) and found that the least costly one (currently at $29.77) is just perfect. View the site and see all the models in order to compare. Kmart and exercise equipment stores also carry minitrampolines; however, I note that my $29.77 model from Walmart is often priced much higher elsewhere.

CLEAR Scoliosis Institute's whole body vibration unit: The Vibe (www.vibeforhealth.com).
Soloflex (www.soloflex.com) **Whole Body Vibration** unit.
THESE ARE TWO ENTIRELY DIFFERENT UNITS IN BOTH THEIR DIMENSIONS AND APPLICATIONS. The Vibe is the unit recommended by CLEAR, and one stands erect on it as it is a round footprint. Soloflex is forty inches long by ten inches wide by five inches high and allows certain exercises to be done while on it. The pricing is vastly different due to different production, mechanisms, and uses.

New Chapter Wholemega Fish Oil. From Swanson or Vitacost, to purchase at a discount. Sign up for e-mails and coupons: www.newchapter.com.

Honey: Y.S. Bee Farm *Raw* Organic Honey. I purchase from both Swanson (discounted) and The Vitamin Shoppe. One can wipe lip of jar with cloth or sponge *barely* damp with warm water; then dry with paper towel to prevent stickiness.

Amber Gargle: I buy the CVS house brand. Some sales during year. Get CVS e-mails.

George's "Always Active®" Aloe (100% Aloe Vera): It is the consistency of water and is delicious. I buy it discounted from Vitacost in the 128 fl. oz. size. I transfer it into a very small bottle to carry outside home as needed. Item #GEO 7100985. (Health Nuts also sells this.)

Elizabeth Arden Flawless Finish pressed cream compact makeup. I buy this at Lord & Taylor and Macy's. It is available at many fine stores.

Rubber glove, fleece lined. I buy this in Waldbaum's supermarket. House brand. Such gloves are available in other markets and drugstores.
Surgical rubber gloves: Very thin, usually sold in boxes with as few as fifteen pair to as many as one hundred; in surgical supply stores, Home Depot (www.homedepot.com), Lowe's (www.lowes.com), and some drugstores. Check prices for best value and various colors.

Escoda brushes from **Jerry's Artarama** (www.jerrysartarama.com), which I use for eyeliner: Kolinsky—Tajmir 1212 0 and Kolinsky—Tajmir 1212 5/0 from Spain.
Yasutomo Y&C Detail Master round brush (www.yasutomo.com) for my eyeliner: DMR 0230 from Japan. Both companies provide wonderful customer service.

Oak Knoll Goats' Milk: I buy this in New York at Whole Foods (www.oakknolldairy.com). I have never drunk more delicious milk!

Organic Valley *Cultured* Butter in Whole Foods (www.organicvalley.coop). Sign up for their newsletters. Get coupons. Products produced without antibiotics, synthetic hormones, or toxic pesticides! *Cultured* **butter** contains healthful microbial cultures.

Alvarado Street Bakery bread (www.alvaradostreetbakery.com), sprouted breads which I buy in New York at Stop & Shop, Whole Foods, Waldbaums, and Health Nuts.

Pete And Gerry's Organic Eggs (www.peteandgerrys.com). I buy in Stop & Shop. A joy!

Normal saline solution, 0.9% Sodium Chloride Irrigation USP in a 500 mL bottle. In New York, I need a prescription for this (because, evidently, drug users need it [as told to me by a pharmacist]). It can be purchased in any pharmacy with a prescription.

Venous insufficiency and circulation products: Swanson, Vitacost, and Puritan's sites and telephones are listed previously. All have frequent sales and sometimes free shipping.
Here is www.standardprocess.com:
Standard Process: **Vasculin, Circuplex, Cataplex B, Cardio-Plus:** These are available from health providers who sell Standard Process (and many sell at a discount).
My source for **ordering Standard Process products is www.drruthcohen.com**. I look up my product numbers on the Standard Process website and e-mail Dr. Ruth (at her chiropractic center). She places my order which is shipped from Standard Process directly to me. Dr. Bruce West (www.healthalertstore.com) also sells these products as do other health-care providers. **Check prices before ordering** as they vary amongst sellers.

Swanson: **DiosVein** (SWU720); **Grapeseed, Green Tea & Pine Bark Complex** (SW1024).
Vitacost: **Horse Chestnut** (NSI 3005796).
Puritan's Pride: **Grape Extract.** Sales frequently including buy one get *two* more free. Also buy one get one free. Puritan's Pride sales change regularly (as do the other companies).

Standard Process: The articles clearly describe each product and how I use it. The products for **colds and respiratory distress**: **Congaplex** (#2925); **Immuplex** (#4960), which is also for **general health support**. For sleep issues: **Cruciferous Complete** (#2960); and **Min-Tran** (#5625) to support **emotional balance and sleep**. Some products offer various-sized bottles. **Cataplex A-C-P** (#0750) for general health, vascular integrity, and immune support; **Cyrtua Plus** (#3330) supports capillary integrity and function and healthy peripheral circulation. **Collagen C** (#2690, 90 count) provides a whole-food source of vitamin C; supports healthy connective tissues and normal immune response.

Standard Process for **stress and adrenal fatigue**: Drenamin (#3700, 360 count).

Standard Process for **digestion** (both are available in small or large bottles): **A-F Betafood** (#0825, 360 count), **Zypan** (#8475, 90 count).

I wrote in various articles that **Standard Process** products are **whole food-based**. Note that one can tell this is true as tablets are slightly different in shading from shipment to shipment because they are formulated from a food base as opposed to standardized synthetic supplements, which are uniformly one color, and labels read "Take with food", which means that food is needed in order to make the supplement more complete. The same point exists for food-based **NutriBiotic** Grapefruit Seed Extract, which has a very mild taste (like grapefruit squeezed into water) that can vary from bottle to bottle as it is based upon the grapefruit product.

B vitamins: Aside from the **B vitamins from Standard Process** (SP) mentioned previously (Vasculin, Cataplex B, Cardio-Plus), there is a B complex from **Puritan's Pride**, but it is not whole food-based: Complete B (item #1250). It is considerably lower in cost than SP, is balanced, and can be used (to save money) instead of or alternately with SP: two weeks SP, for example, and two weeks Complete B. Take one caplet two or three times daily with meals and with good fats in the stomach.

Vitamin C from Puritan's Pride and considerably lower cost than Standard Process as it is not whole food-based (#430, 500 mg). Sales throughout the year. Sign up for e-mails.

Compression hose: www.compressionsale.com, 800-504-7315; www.discountsurgical.com, 800-982-0939; and www.foryourlegs.com, 877-846-4600.

JCPenney (www.jcp.com) pantyhose, both *support* and *plain*.
Product: East 5th Sheer Caress Sheerest Support **Pantyhose**. They have a beautiful, silky sheen and durability. The hose is also available without the support factor. There are sales all the time. Superb value.

Gold's Horseradish: I buy this at Stop & Shop supermarket where it is always priced well. It is widely available in many stores in white, red (from fresh beets), and hot.

Full-spectrum natural lighting and bulbs: www.verilux.com is where I buy all my bulbs and special lamps. Sign up for e-mails. Sales throughout the year. I have also bought full-spectrum tube bulbs for my office ceiling from **www.lowes.com** and **www.homedepot.com**.

Jay Robb Chocolate Whey Protein is available from Swanson, Vitacost, and The Vitamin Shoppe in several size bags and prices. One can also order directly from Jay Robb and get the best price with automatic monthly shipments (www.jayrobb.com). Several flavors. (877-529-7622) As I wrote, I mix chocolate with Oak Knoll Goats' Milk.

"Jay Robb Non-GMO Chocolate Whey Protein Isolate powder is made from the finest natural ingredients and delivers twenty-five grams of first class protein, 0-fat, 0-cholesterol, 0-sugars, and only 1 gram of carbohydrate per 30 gram serving. Only cold-processed cross-flow microfiltered whey protein isolate is used as the protein source, and this material comes from farm-raised, pasture-grazed, grass-fed cows not treated with the synthetic bovine growth hormone rBGH.

"Whey protein isolate, used exclusively in Jay Robb's Whey Protein, is created by microfiltering liquid whey through a special ceramic membrane to create the highest grade of whey protein. This unique process also yields a whey protein isolate that is much higher in protein than a whey protein concentrate and is also rich in immunoglobulins, alpha-lactalbumin, and beta-lactoalbumin and other immune boosting factors.

"BEWARE of most protein powders on the market! Many formulas contain cheaper proteins, massive amounts of SUGAR, and refined carbohydrates in the form of: FRUCTOSE, GLUCOSE, GLUCOSE POLYMERS, MALTODEXTRIN, as well as fake sugars chemically developed, such as ASPARTAME, SUCRALOSE, ACESULFAME-K, and POLYDEXTROSE, just to name a few." **READ LABELS!!**

Living Nutz (www.livingnutz.com) for raw organic nuts (207-780-1101) including **un**pasteurized!! Very nice folks in Maine. So kind and reliable. Great gifts. Sales throughout year.

Index

A

acid reflux, 43, 62, 65
acid suppressant, 65
acne, 23, 25, 141
adrenal fatigue, 178
A-F Betafood, 66, 178
aftershave, 108
age spots, 29-30
alfalfa, 120, 134, 136, 173
almonds, unpasteurized, 88, 127, 179
aloe. *See* George's "Always Active®" Aloe
Alvarado Street Bakery bread, 88, 176
Alzheimer's disease, 75
animals. *See* veterinarian products
antibacterial soap and wipes, 150, 154
arms
    isometrics, 70-72
    underarm flab toning, 67-68
arrhythmias, 15, 78, 82, 138
arthritis, 34, 36, 97-98
astigmatism, 158

B

baby potties, 115-16
backache, 55, 111
bacteria, 19, 31, 47-50, 83, 85-86, 93, 132, 138, 156
baking, 126-27. *See also* coconut oil
balance, 33, 47, 74, 76, 95, 99, 120-21, 142-43, 145, 177
bandage, 18-19

bee propolis, 121, 136, 173
belching, 62, 65
betaine hydrochloride, 65-66
Betaine Plus, 65-67
bioflavonoids, 36-37
bio-identical hormone replacement therapy, 15
bladder, 115-16, 134-36
bleeding, 48, 137-38, 173
bloating, 42-43, 62
blood pressure, 95, 113, 122
body movements, shoulders and posture, 31-32, 34, 37, 40, 56
bowel, 13, 61, 66, 115-18
brain function, cross crawl, 74
Brazil nuts, 127
bread, 18, 67, 87-88
    Alvarado Street Bakery, 88, 176
bromelain, 137-38
buffing skin, 105-6
burn marks, 29
burns, 20-21
bustline, 70-71
buttock, wiping tips, 29, 118

C

calcium, 37, 50, 58, 79-81, 145-46, 172
calories, 46, 77, 139
cancer, 15, 43, 116, 139, 154, 160-61, 165
Caprobiotics Plus+, 49
caraway seeds, 66-67
Cardio-Plus, 82, 147, 177-78

181

cardiovascular workout, 78
cashew nuts, 88, 127
Cataplex B, 82, 147, 177-78
Celtic Sea Salt, 94-96, 127, 130, 134, 172
cervical dysplasia, 12, 158-61, 163-64, 166
charcoal, 140, 142, 173
cheek blush, 104
chest constriction, 140-41
chilling quickly, wine or any beverage, 142
cholesterol, 125-26, 139, 148, 179
chopsticks, 97-98
Christmas trees, 156
circulation, 16-17, 32, 54, 106-7, 111-12, 146-48, 150, 177
Circuplex, 147, 177
coconut oil, 22-26, 29-30, 86, 101-3, 106, 125-27, 171. *See also* oil
colds, 93, 128, 132, 134, 142, 150-51, 177
collagen, 137-38, 165, 177
cologne, 20, 108
Complete B, 82, 178
compression hose, 149-50, 178
constipation, 43, 115-16
cooking, 126. *See also* Celtic Sea Salt; coconut oil
coordination, 74-75
coughs, 78-79, 128, 132, 134-35, 142, 146, 150-51
cracks, heel, 13, 122-24
crooked penis, 28
cross crawl, 74-77
cryosurgery, 161-62
cuts, 83
  paper, 83-84, 89
CVS, 103, 108, 133, 174-75

D

dandruff, 13, 22, 125, 142
deep breathing, 35, 55, 59, 86-87
dehydration, symptom, 21, 118
derrières, wiping tips, 29, 118
diarrhea, 62, 65
diet, 22, 28, 42, 44, 46, 80, 84, 115, 123, 158, 164-66
digestive problems, 42
DiosVein, 16, 147-48, 177
diversity, 168
Douglas Laboratories, 65, 79-80, 172
drinking water, 12, 19
dust mites, 155

E

ear pressure, 110
Echinacea, 128-29, 132, 173
eggs, 45, 126-27, 171, 176
elbow, funny bone injury (isometrics for), 70-72
elimination, 63-64, 115-17
emu oil, 22-27, 29, 85, 101-3, 109-10, 118, 148, 171-72
English muffin, 20
enzymes, 84, 119, 123, 135
  digestive, 42, 61-63
  healing, 84, 94, 119
  pancreatic, 65
exercises, 58, 67-68, 71-72, 75, 175
  arm, 55-56, 68
  isometric, 35, 111
  neck, 56
expressions, 38

extended life span, 43
eye shadow, 104, 114

F

fats, 22, 45-47, 58, 81, 122-23, 125, 140
  dietary, 66
  good, 28, 44-45, 81, 123, 125-27, 178
  healthy, 126
  incorrect, 81
  trans, 45
fatty acids, 122
feces. *See* stool
fiber, 64, 117-18
financial tips/articles, 166-70
fingernails, 22, 29, 31, 62, 145, 149
fish oil, 121-22, 138, 142, 165, 175
flashlight, 52-53, 144
flax oil and seeds, 81, 88, 126, 171
Flax-Orange Handmade Bath Soap, 30
flexibility, 168
floss/floss sticks, 48, 94, 96, 172
fluoride, 12, 16, 26, 87, 94, 99, 139
folate, 161-62, 165, 174
food combining, 28, 42-44, 62-64, 118, 127, 164
food poisoning, 139-40
frowning, 39, 138
fruits, 28, 36, 42-43, 46, 63-64, 115, 118, 124, 147, 150, 154, 164
full-spectrum lighting, 157-58
funny bone, 33, 42, 70, 72
fur, 89
Future Sticks chopsticks, 97-98, 172

G

gardening, 155
gargle, 51, 94, 97, 129-30, 133-35, 175
garlic, 129, 132, 138, 142, 173
gas, 42-43, 62, 65, 73, 98, 113, 152, 161
George's "Always Active®" Aloe (100% Aloe Vera), 20, 51, 109-10, 133, 136-37, 176
germs, 31, 89, 93, 98, 128, 150-51
gingivitis, 47
gloves, surgical and rubber, 18, 25, 29, 53, 88-89, 148-49, 176
glycerin soap, 16, 30, 94, 106, 173
goat's milk, 50
Gold's Horseradish, 179
Good-Gums, 16, 48-49, 93-97, 172
growth hormone
  bovine, 179
  human (in urine), 83
GUM PerioBalance, 47-49, 95, 172
gymnasium, 55, 174

H

hair
  dryer, 19, 128
  follicles, 26
  regrowth, 26
hand tremors, 98
hangover, 139, 142
hang upside down, 54, 70, 159
Health Nuts, 127, 136, 172, 176. *See also* George's "Always Active®" Aloe (100% Aloe Vera)
hearing, 19, 131, 156, 159, 169
heartburn, 62, 65

heart disease, 15, 78, 82, 122
heart flutter, 15, 78-79
hemorrhoids, 16, 29, 116, 146, 148
herbs, 28, 120, 135-36, 138, 146
hives, 83-84, 148
holistic medicine, 15
Home Depot, 18, 89, 158, 176, 179
honey, 23, 47, 117, 121, 129-30, 134-37, 140, 171, 175
Horse Chestnut, 148, 177
horseradish, 19, 139, 142, 179
Horsetail, 138, 173
hotel tip (wash the glasses), 150-51
hot flashes, 86-87, 120-21
human growth hormone, in our urine, 83
humming, 51-52
hydrochloric acid, 61-63
hydrogen peroxide, 3 percent, 19, 85, 90-91, 93, 96-97, 133, 155-56

I

icing wine or beverage quickly, 142
inflammation, 46-48, 95, 121-22, 137-38, 149
injuries, 110
insect bites, 83-84
insomnia, 143
invert, 54, 57-58, 62
investing, 166-69
isometrics, 33, 42, 68-72, 111, 116, 144, 150

J

Jay Robb Chocolate Whey Protein, 51, 179
JCPenney, 106, 150, 174, 178

Jerry's Artarama, 114, 176
jewelry, 19, 135
Juvéderm, 173

K

King Juan Carlos, tea, 152
Kyolic Garlic, 129, 132, 142, 173

L

legume, 120
lighting, 157-58, 179
Lipanase, 65
lipstick, 21, 52, 90, 104-5, 108
liver, 66, 100, 113, 139, 145
Living Nutz, 127, 179
Lord & Taylor, 176
lotion, self-tanning, 88
Lowe's, 18, 89, 158, 176, 179
low-fat diet, danger of, 123, 125
lozenge, 47-49, 130
lubricant, 22-23

M

Maca, 120-21, 174
Macy's, 176
magnesium, 37, 58, 79-80, 146, 172
makeup, 18, 25, 38, 99, 101-4, 108-9, 176
  applying, 18, 101-2
  base, 103, 109
  brushes, 108, 114
  eye, 25, 108, 111, 114
  face, 26
  removing, 25-26, 101-2, 106
massage, 24-25, 32
Maybelline, 104-5

McNulty's, New York, 152-53
memory, 39, 45, 54, 74-75, 96
memory loss, short-term, 54
mental agility/stability, 74
    cross crawl for brain/memory and physical help, 74-77
milk, 19, 50-51, 80, 173, 176, 179
    cow, 50-51
    goat, 45, 49-51, 81, 126-27, 153
    mother's, 50
minitrampoline, 72-73, 76, 175
moisturizers, 22, 24, 101, 106, 108, 114
moles, 96-97, 138
Mt. Capra, 49, 172

N

nail polish, 20, 89, 91-92, 105, 118-19, 174
nails, 13, 18, 20, 31, 65, 88-89, 93, 118, 145
nervous system, 75-76, 125
newsletters, 11, 13-14, 17, 34, 171, 176
NK Tea Salon, Stockholm, 152-53
nodules, 136-37
normal saline solution, 132, 177
nose spray, 13, 15
NutriBiotic, 19, 86, 91, 129, 132-33, 138, 154, 173, 178
NutriBiotic Grapefruit Seed Extract, 19, 86, 129, 132-33, 138, 154, 173, 178
nuts, 81, 125, 127, 179

O

Oak Knoll Goats' Milk, 51, 81, 126, 176, 179
oil
    emu, 22-27, 29, 85, 101-3, 109-10, 118, 148, 171
    fish, 121-22, 138, 142, 165, 175
    jojoba, 101-2, 174
    organic coconut, 23, 30, 45, 81, 126, 171
    organic virgin coconut, 22, 25-27, 29-31, 49, 86, 101-2, 106, 171
Olive Leaf Extract, 129, 174
Omega Nutrition, 22, 25, 27, 30, 49, 86, 101, 106, 126-27, 142, 154, 171
    Flax-Orange Handmade Bath Soap, 30
    liquid soap, 106, 154, 171
    Natural Face & Body Soap, 30
    Organic Coconut Oil, 30, 126
    Organic Unfiltered Apple Cider Vinegar, 142
    Organic Virgin Coconut Oil, 22, 25, 27, 30, 49, 86, 101, 127
    See also coconut oil
Organic Valley Cultured Butter, 88, 126, 171, 176
Osteo-guard, 79-80, 172
osteoporosis, 78, 80
overdose (of supplements), 124, 139
ozone therapy, 165-66

P

PABA, 27-28, 174
Pacific Place tea, Honolulu, 152-53
packing, 18, 89, 151

pain, 20-21, 29, 31-32, 34, 41, 57, 70, 113, 139
   back, 57, 65
   chest, 140
   hip, 33-34
   joint, 110
   lower back, 13, 16, 57
   muscle, 110
   neck, 41
palpitations, 13, 15, 37, 58, 78, 138, 146
pantyhose, 18, 92, 106-7, 119, 149-50, 178
Pap smear, 160, 165-66
Parkinson's, 98
Pau d'Arco, 128
pecans, 88, 127
penis, crooked/curved, 28
penis lubrication, 22-23
perfume, 20, 108
periodontal disease, 47-48, 95
periodontitis, 47-48
peristalsis, 46, 88, 115, 118
peroxide. *See* hydrogen peroxide, 3 percent
pesticides, 14, 51, 126, 176
Pete And Gerry's Organic Eggs, 176
petroleum jelly, 20, 108
pets, nutrition. *See* veterinarian products
Peyronie's disease, crooked/curved penis, 28
pillows, 155
pimples, 19, 138
pistachio nuts, 127
plant care/watering, 155-56
poisoning, 129, 139-40, 142
posture, 20, 31-32, 34, 37, 40, 42, 56
potatoes, 42, 63, 126, 171

prebiotics, 50
pregnant, tips, 67, 107, 128
prescription drugs, 11, 13, 81, 126
probiotics, 47-50, 95, 172
   oral, 47-49
Prodentis, 47-48
pulling (for gum health), 47-49, 94
pumpkin seeds, 88, 121, 127
   for hot flashes, 121
Puritan's Pride, 30, 82, 106, 136, 140, 148, 173-74, 177-78

R

rashes, 31, 43, 83-85, 106, 131-32, 141, 148
rebounder (minitrampoline), 73-74, 76-77, 175
recorking, 143
rectal irritation, 148
respiratory distress, 177
restless legs, 143, 146
Retin-A, 19, 85-86
Revlon, 104
Rimmel, 104
roasting food, 126-27
rosacea, 25, 83, 85, 132, 141

S

saliva, 44, 48-49, 66, 84, 94, 118-19
salt. *See* Selina Naturally
saute' onions, 127
scoliosis, 40-41, 70-71, 175
seeds, 66, 81, 125, 127
Selina Naturally, 16, 49, 94-96, 127, 130, 132, 134, 142, 172
September 11, *53*, *132*, *167*
sex, 22, 164

sinuses, 13, 73, 95, 131-32
slant board, 54, 58, 63, 68-69, 86, 115, 159
sleep, in total darkness, 52-53, 113-14
sleeping positions, 111
Soloflex, 33, 175
"Source List," 171-79
spider veins, 106-8, 147
spine, elongate, 31-33, 37, 39
stability (mental and physical), regained with cross crawl, 76
stomach, 20, 33-35, 37, 42-44, 46-47, 54, 56-59, 61-67, 72, 80, 87, 118, 120, 123, 125, 139-42, 162, 178
stool, 21, 64, 115-18
Stop & Shop, 176, 179. *See also* Gold's Horseradish; Pete And Gerry's Organic Eggs
stress, 28, 35, 57, 122, 144-45, 149, 156-57, 178
stroke, 104, 108-9, 121-22
sunflower seeds, 88, 127
Sunstar Americas Inc, 172
supplements, 11, 13-15, 17, 28, 58, 64-65, 75, 80, 82, 120, 123, 128-31, 140, 144, 146, 148, 157-58, 161, 164-65, 171, 178
Swanson, 101, 122-23, 125, 136, 145, 147-48, 172-75, 177, 179
Swanson Grapeseed, Green Tea & Pine Bark Complex, 148
symptom, 13, 15-16, 21, 37, 41, 62, 65, 75, 82, 95-96, 118, 125, 157, 161

T

Te & Kaffi, Iceland, 152-53
tea, 19, 21, 29, 50, 80, 141, 145, 151-53, 177
  decaffeinated, 153
  loose leaf, 151-53
teddy bears, 155
Thayers Slippery Elm Lozenges, 52, 130, 172
thighs
  isometrics, 150
  in stair climbing, 78
  toning, 146, 150
Thunder Ridge Emu Oil, 22, 101, 172
thyroid gland, 24, 101-2
timing, 168
T.J. Maxx, 106, 174
toast, 20, 81, 88, 171
  Alvarado Street Bakery, 88
toning, 58, 67-68, 72, 75, 77-78, 114, 136, 150
toothbrush, 16, 30, 58, 93-94, 97, 151
toothpicks, 19, 96
Total Gym, 54, 159, 174-75
travelling, 114, 150

U

underarm flab, 67
urination, 134, 136
urine (healing enzymes; human growth hormone), 19, 83-86, 109-10, 119

V

vaginal dryness, 22
vaginal lubrication, 22
vaginal maintenance, 24
Vasculin, 82, 146-47, 177-78
vegetables, 28, 42, 46, 63, 118, 125, 145, 150, 154, 164
Vegetarian Enzyme, 65-66
veins, 16, 147-48
  spider, 106-8, 147
  varicose, 106-7, 147
venous insufficiency, 16, 82, 111-12, 146-49, 177
Verilux, 158, 179
veterinarian products (from Standard Process), 130-31
viruses, 43, 49, 93
visualization, 58
Vitacost, 80, 101, 109, 122-23, 136, 148, 172-77, 179
vitamin, 28, 79, 140, 163
  A, 122-25, 161-62, 165, 174
  B, 81-82
  C, 37, 147, 164-65, 177-78
  D, 16, 55, 57-58, 71, 79-81, 126
  D3, 16, 55, 57-58, 79
  E, 125, 138
  K, 80, 145
  K2, 11, 37, 58, 79-81, 138
Vitamin Shoppe, 91, 101, 125, 172-73, 175, 179
Vitex, 121, 174
vocal cords, 20, 51-52, 136-37
voice, 51-52, 105, 137
  overused, 51, 133, 136
  strained, 51, 136

W

Waldbaum's supermarket, 176
Walgreens, 96, 104, 108, 172, 174. *See also* floss sticks; Wet n' Wild
walking
  backward, 75, 77
  forward, 77
Walmart, 74, 175
walnuts, 88, 127
water
  distilled, 59-61, 88, 99-100, 109, 156
  drinking. *See* drinking water
weight, 42-46, 50, 68, 74, 78, 100
weight loss, 43-44, 78
Wet n' Wild, 104-5, 108, 174
whole body vibration, 31, 33, 175
whole food, 14-15, 75, 81, 130-31, 146, 165, 178
Whole Foods, 127, 176. *See also* Oak Knoll Goats' Milk; Organic Valley Cultured Butter
wine, 45, 90, 124, 142-43, 151, 164
wiping tips for tushies (adult and children), 29
wrinkles, 38-39, 111, 137-38, 173

Z

zinc, 22, 123
Zypan, 66-67, 178

Author's Biography

Starting from Carole Lynn Steiner's early adulthood, "Mybyble" is the compilation of her lifetime experience accumulating and developing information that is simple to use, direct, and easy to adapt to individual, everyday needs. These are many of the things that make Carole Lynn's life easier and give the author control over what happens to her. There are even life-saving tips and financial tips! One will want to refer back to articles in "Mybyble", many of which are so understandable that one says: "Why didn't *I* think of that?" Carole Lynn has put them all under one cover.

Carole Lynn has been a 'life coach' to some . . . . helping them recognize and change or improve habits and life styles. Regarding the health information, she has taught this to many people who say that they owe their improved lives to the author. After Carole Lynn graduated from New York University, she became associated with the fifth largest medical center in the metropolitan New York area. Initially, she was involved in Business & Financial Development including obtaining government grants for the medical center's many divisions; however, the Director of the medical center agreed with her suggestion that they should publish a health newsletter, and he tapped Carole Lynn to do it! This time it paid to volunteer!

Thus, the author became the founder, writer, and editor of a very successful international, comprehensive health newsletter which was published bi-monthly, with each issue covering health, sex, exercise, and diet. It caught the eye of the president of the largest radio station in New York at that time, and Carole Lynn furnished the station with a broad range of health tips. That segued, in a short period of time, into health segments on a major television network news program.

Carole Lynn is accustomed to speaking in front of large audiences including in person, on radio, and on television. She has given radio interviews as well as doing financial segments for Bloomberg radio and has been interviewed on television and radio both domestically and internationally. Carole Lynn has also spoken to groups of up to 2,300 for a major international brokerage firm and for private industry.

While the international business world is Carole Lynn Steiner's occupational domain, health and better living are her private concerns. Please refer to "Mybyble" in order to help improve your daily life as well as for health issues. It contains a comprehensive compendium of usable tips including health, sex, exercise, diet, and financial. "Cough for Heart Flutters", "Urine Heals Paper Cuts", "Use A Small Hair Blower for Sniffles", "Back Pain", and "Food Combining for Good Digestion, Health, and Weight Loss" will be tips that can be used throughout your life and shared with others, and you will hear what the author has heard so many times: "Wow! I don't believe it. You should write a book!"

Carole Lynn wrote "Mybyble" as though she was the reader. Hence, there is a really comprehensive Index as well as multiple headings above each article regarding subject matter. Being the 'face behind the cover' is a serious undertaking.

Find just a few tips that make you happy, and you are rewarded forever. Some months from now, you will suddenly think: What was that article in "Mybyble"?, and you can take pleasure in the ease of quickly looking up what **you** need.

Health and habits are a commitment. You can spend your days later in life commiserating over lost opportunities while running to doctors' offices for tests, shots, and prescriptions, OR, you can gain confidence and take control of what you can do for yourself. **Carole Lynn personally has been more than repaid (over these many years** from her reading and research) with a healthier: back, gums, circulation, total health, confidence in the knowledge that she gains, and much more. **The author believes that you can use "Mybyble" to your benefit in the same way. Any great tip which lasts a lifetime allows the reader to reap a great reward** . . . . and "Mybyble" has many such tips all in one slender digest.

Everything in "Mybyble" is an opening. These are life tips . . . . things that you can use every day. They become second nature . . . . and make your life better. From Carole Lynn to you: "I wish you well."